diary of an
ALZHEIMER'S
CAREGIVER

diary of an
ALZHEIMER'S
CAREGIVER

Robert
Hershberger

Purdue University Press · West Lafayette, Indiana

Cataloging-in-Publication Data is available from the Library of Congress.

978-1-61249-734-1 (print)
978-1-61249-735-8 (epub)
978-1-61249-736-5 (epdf)

Cover background image: iStock.com/voyata

In loving memory of
Rev. Deanna (Dee) Hershberger

Contents

Preface and Acknowledgments

THIS BOOK PROVIDES AN UP CLOSE AND PERSONAL VIEW OF DEANNA (Dee) Hershberger's four-and-a-half-year journey through Alzheimer's disease, from its first manifestations in the fall of 2010 until her death on March 1, 2015. As Dee's husband of more than fifty years and her primary caregiver, I first recorded changes as they occurred but later as an almost daily diary. I hope that this digest of the original entries will help readers appreciate what occurred throughout the course of the disease.

During the first two years, Dee gradually lost her short-term memory but maintained most of her physical and social abilities. The last two years became an excruciating ordeal for Dee and an emotional roller coaster for me as she lost her long-term memory, experienced psychotic episodes, had uncontrollable violent behavior, lost physical abilities, became incontinent, and suffered from undetected illnesses.

This journey can happen to anyone—either as the person with the disease or as the primary caregiver. The yearly reflections and advice to caregivers shared in this book should interest affected family members, medical personnel, psychologists, church members, ministers, deacons, and those in families with a history of Alzheimer's disease. It will help all readers appreciate the emotional and financial consequences of the disease, as well as what to do and what not to do about extremely difficult behavior when caring for a loved one with Alzheimer's.

The book ends with photos spanning Dee's life, including the decades we spent together, celebrating all she meant to me and everyone around her before contracting the disease.

I WISH TO ACKNOWLEDGE MY DEAR DECEASED DEANNA FOR THE BRAVE battle she undertook in 2010. I also wish to express my gratitude to the following people for helping me during the course of Dee's disease: my sister Louise Clarke, brother Edward, sons Vernon and Andrew, and their spouses and families; Glenn and Carolyn Bradley; many members of Payson United Methodist Church, especially Marcina Brook, Joyce and Larry Kennedy, and Chris Spencer, for providing important emotional support; and Dr. Alan Michels, his nurse practitioners, and several part-time caregivers for providing medical and caregiving support.

I would also like to acknowledge my sister Louise and Sandra Carver for helping me reduce the manuscript length, as well as Justin Race, Jan Dougherty, Dr. Richard Caselli, Diane Mockbee, and two anonymous reviewers for the Purdue University Press for their thoughtful suggestions for improving the contents and encouraging publication of the diary. I also appreciate very much the editorial, design, and marketing support provided by Katherine Purple, Kelley Kimm, Chris Brannan, and Bryan Shaffer of the Purdue University Press.

Many thanks to all of you.

Robert Hershberger
January 2022

1

First Year
of the Journey

ॐ

IT BEGAN WITH SUCH INNOCENCE.

"Honey, what is that green stuff in the refrigerator?"

"I don't know. Show me."

She opened the refrigerator, pulled out the hydrator, pointed at the celery.

"Honey, that's celery. You know what that is."

"Yes, I do now. But each time I look at it, I can't remember its name."

"Well, Sweetheart, you know it now."

"Yes, I do. Wonderful! It's . . . I can't remember."

"Celery, silly. You are such a wonderful person. You'll remember it now."

"It's . . . No I don't remember! It's not silly. It's awful!"

"Celery!"

"Celery, celery, celery, celery, celery. Now I'll remember."

But she didn't. The word was lost. Never to return.

SEPTEMBER–DECEMBER 2010 ❧

After a heavy late summer rainstorm, Dee and I discovered water all over the floor in an office where we volunteered. She and another volunteer carried fallen gypsum board to a dumpster in the alley, unaware of the black mold on the back side of the board. Shortly thereafter, the other person had serious respiratory problems relating to the mold that required extensive medical treatment and recuperation time. Dee experienced no respiratory problems but could not remember familiar words such as celery, asparagus, and fork, among others. We wondered if the mold affected her memory, but her doctor felt that Dee's memory loss might relate to a thyroid imbalance noted on a previous examination. The doctor increased a naturopathic supplement called Raw Thyroid from two to four pills a day and put Dee on Aricept, a memory medication.

Dee maintained a positive attitude but expressed concern about the mold and her loss of some words. We enjoyed social occasions with friends from our church, a political organization, and Amnesty International. We also enjoyed bicycling, playing tennis, and golfing together. Dee continued taking a yoga class at the community college and taught yoga to several women at our church. We celebrated Thanksgiving with our youngest son and his family in Ohio. No one mentioned Dee's trouble finding familiar words.

JANUARY–MARCH 2011 ❧

Dee found it hard to remember more words. She had difficulty balancing the family checkbook, something she had easily accomplished ever since we married. She became increasingly frustrated with her computer, finding it both uncooperative and difficult to operate. She became short tempered and began to lose weight. I wondered if either the mold or Raw Thyroid had gotten into her brain and caused both the memory problems and weight loss.

After another visit, Dee's doctor referred her to a neuropsychologist in Phoenix for a memory test. Dee returned to the waiting room irritated with the doctor's manner and the repetitiveness of the questions. The examination showed that Dee had mildly impaired memory and cognitive abilities and the doctor recommended that she not continue to drive. This advice upset Dee so much that she discounted both his analysis and conclusions.

Dee's primary care doctor then increased the dosage of Raw Thyroid from four to five pills a day. However, after I read a label warning against taking more than one Raw Thyroid pill a day, I insisted that Dee heed this warning. I also made an appointment with a neurologist at the University of Arizona Medical Center to seek better advice on how to treat Dee's condition.

We continued to bicycle several times a week and went skiing with friends. Dee showed no signs of impairment with either activity and kept driving in Payson and on short trips to the Phoenix area. We also took a splendid bicycling trip with good friends from California to see Arches National Park in southern Utah. They did not notice Dee's problem finding words.

APRIL–MAY 2011 ❧

Dee's memory problems got worse. More words failed to come when she needed them, and she often forgot where she put things. She could not spell familiar words or remember practically anything just discussed.

Dee accused me of not listening to her one day and insisted that we see a psychologist to sort out our communication difficulties. I felt we had few problems and could sort them out by ourselves but reluctantly agreed. After listening to our stories, the psychologist concluded that the communication problem existed mostly in Dee's mind. She suggested that Dee listen better to me. This recommendation did not please Dee, but thereafter she said little about my not listening to her. At other times she would assert, "You're trying to drive me crazy." She also threatened suicide. This concerned me a lot, so I began to hide objects she could use to kill herself.

One day Dee told me that a man she talked with on her daily walks invited her to have lunch with him. She could or would not identify the man, so I advised her strongly not to accept his invitation. I eventually concluded that he existed only in her imagination. Perhaps it was her way to determine if I really love her. More often she suggested that we should divorce, saying, "You'll be better off without me."

"I don't want a divorce. I want to live with you," I repeatedly responded.

Even if Dee could cover up her memory difficulties with friends and relatives, her memory loss clearly disturbed her and upset me. I knew that some form of dementia, possibly caused by the mold or thyroid imbalance, was resulting in memory problems that we would have to live with unless we could discover the cause and remove it.

While Dee experienced these changes in her capabilities, we began to plan and execute a yearlong celebration of our fiftieth wedding anniversary. This helped to distract us from our marital difficulties. We agreed to visit all the places where we lived since our marriage and to travel to Alaska, a place we had dreamed about visiting for years.

We traveled first to San Francisco, the city where we lived during our first year of marriage. We visited our two apartments and other places we remembered. We socialized with a number of old friends and no one seemed to notice Dee's memory difficulties. We enjoyed the experience.

We also made plans to visit my hometown, Pocatello, Idaho, where Dee and I spent the second through fourth years of our marriage. My brother, sister, and I made arrangements for a family reunion in midsummer to celebrate our parents' lives in Pocatello.

JUNE–JULY 2011 ॐ

Dee and I continued to practice yoga, hike, bike, fish, and play golf and tennis. We also enjoyed social occasions with friends. She remained in good spirits, and her earlier concerns about divorce or suicide subsided. We led the good life and looked forward to our planned trips.

We took turns driving to Pocatello for the family reunion in early July and enjoyed visiting with our extended family and many friends. We especially enjoyed recalling how Dee got to know and love my parents while we lived in Pocatello. We shared memories about our two jobs, attending church, going on short trips, and having dinners with my parents and other friends.

After the family reunion, our nuclear family drove to Grand Teton National Park and visited the places where Dee and I fell in love and agreed to marry. "Grandma Dee" scurried around in seventh heaven with her children and grandchildren in this wonderful place. Unfortunately, when we returned home she had no memory of these times. Her short-term memory had vanished.

We visited the neurologist at University Medical Center in late July. He had reviewed all of Dee's records and talked to her at great length. He doubted that mold caused the memory loss and said that Dee should stop taking Raw Thyroid. He suggested that she use an approved thyroid medication to rule out or establish whether thyroid imbalance actually caused her declining mental abilities. Dee liked this doctor and agreed to take his advice, especially because he said nothing about her driving.

I persuaded Dee to see my primary care doctor after this visit because I no longer trusted hers. I think my doctor accepted her as a new patient knowing that taking care of her would also be taking care of me. He did a thorough physical examination of Dee, looked at her medical history, and studied the recent reports. He took her off the Raw Thyroid and prescribed several new medications and tests to rule out or in thyroid imbalance or mold as the cause of Dee's problems.

AUGUST–OCTOBER 2011 ?

Dee took the regimen of medically approved thyroid and mold medications prescribed by her new (my) primary care doctor. Her mood definitely improved and her weight stabilized at ten pounds less than her previous weight. She had gone from a size 10 to a size 8 in just one year. I wondered, and still wonder, if Raw Thyroid at high dosage should be advertised as a weight loss supplement.

Our anniversary celebration continued in August with the long-awaited trip to Alaska. While packing her suitcase the day before the trip, Dee kept putting in and taking out clothes, cosmetics, and the like. She did this late into the evening. This made me very nervous so I got up after she fell asleep to see if she packed everything needed. The suitcase was a mess. I pointed this out to Dee in the morning. Embarrassed, she asked me to repack for her, admitting that packing confused her. I did the repacking, making certain that I packed everything needed for every day of our cruise.

We flew nonstop to Vancouver, British Columbia, where best friends from our year in San Francisco met us. We enjoyed our time together visiting special places in Vancouver. However, when they took us to the dock to board the cruise ship, the husband pulled me aside and asked, "Does Dee have early-stage Alzheimer's disease?" He was the first person to ask this about Dee. He had firsthand experience with relatives with Alzheimer's and recognized some symptoms.

Dee made it clear to me that she did not want me to discuss her memory difficulties with anyone, so I did not. I often wished that I could ask for prayers from people in our church. Instead, I prayed for her swift recovery. In this regard, my religious beliefs, especially regarding prayer, were badly shaken by the lack of any positive answer. I became convinced (and remain so) that unlike during the time when Jesus lived on earth, God no longer intercedes with miracles on behalf of faithful followers like Dee.

We enjoyed the eleven-day cruise up the Inside Passage to Seward and the places along the way. Because Dee could not keep track of her clothes and cosmetics, I appreciated not having to move baggage every day. We loved seeing all the sights, but unfortunately I contracted a version of Alaska crud on the trip so could not drive or fly to Dee's childhood home for her college reunion. However, by then we knew that the rest of our planned anniversary travels would not occur. The confusion caused by travel bothered Dee a lot, and having to remember everything for two wore on me.

NOVEMBER–DECEMBER 2011 ❧

I looked forward to a scheduled visit to see a noted neurologist at the Mayo Clinic to discover the cause of Dee's memory problems and began to think she had Alzheimer's disease.

One Sunday, the new minister at our church asked Dee to help serve communion. Dee had served communion often in the past as an ordained Methodist deacon, but this time she needed a lot of coaching. After the service, the lady who helped Dee asked me, "Does Dee have memory problems?" She was the first person in Payson to bring this up to me. Dee was such a friendly, loving, capable person that most parishioners did not suspect she could no longer fully participate in church activities.

In November, the senior neurologist at the Mayo Clinic introduced us to a young doctor in her last year of residency working with him on Dee's case. We liked them both and felt an answer regarding Dee's memory problems would soon be forthcoming.

"There has been enough trying this and that. It's time to find out what is really going on," the senior physician told us. I liked this approach.

The young doctor gave Dee a battery of language and memory tests similar to those given by the neuropsychologist. She also ordered blood work, brain scans, and everything else that could tell us something.

We ended 2011 in Payson with our entire family in our home just after Christmas. We stayed close to home to enjoy good food, board games, athletic activities, and lots of family togetherness. Dee participated in every activity. It was a special time and a fitting end to our fiftieth wedding anniversary year. No one in the family seemed to realize that Dee had memory problems. And true to Dee's request, I told no one about them.

Reflections on the First Year ❧

Looking back on what I wrote in the first year's diary, I tried to remember if I missed some early signs of the onset of Dee's dementia. Maybe I did. She became very interested in mental exercise shortly after retiring in 2005. She worked every day on crossword puzzles and several books of Sudoku. Was this a sign? Maybe so! If so, she had me fooled.

Reviewing Dee's on-again, off-again diaries from the years before she died, I found no mention before 2010 of any concerns about memory loss. But in January of 2010, just after she visited her doctor in Pine, Dee wrote, "I hope I can keep my mind." She had several similar entries during that spring and summer but said nothing about them to me. She remained engaged in every activity as before and seemed completely happy with her life and me.

So do I have any advice about being more observant for signs of dementia? No, not really. By the time you discover that a loved one has Alzheimer's, it is probably too late to alter the course of the already advanced stage of the disease.

Alzheimer's research is now oriented toward earlier detection of the disease using genetic testing and the like. Research findings may provide an opportunity to catch the disease early enough to stop it from progressing. People with a parent or grandparent who died with or from the disease would be wise to check into early intervention.

Advice to Caregivers ❧

1. Make contingency plans for how to deal with Alzheimer's disease, or any other catastrophic illness or accident, before it happens to you or your loved one. Do you have sufficient financial resources to care for the person at home or in a care facility? Do you have a network of

family and friends willing to support you in caregiving? Can you afford to pay for long-term care insurance? If so, read the policy carefully because many policies have such onerous qualifications that you may have to pay thousands of dollars caring for your loved one before coverage begins. Could you or your loved one qualify for your state's long-term care program? If you are financially strapped, this could help a lot.

2. You and your loved one should stay active, eat well, sleep enough, exercise, socialize, and read a lot to try to forestall or prevent onset of the disease. Be aware, however, that even with these efforts, you or your loved one may still get this or another terrible disease.

3. If it becomes clear that a loved one has Alzheimer's disease or another form of dementia, get your financial affairs in order quickly and simplified to the maximum extent possible. Definitely get your legal and health care directives in order because the time will come when your loved one will be unable to make decisions or even to sign his or her name to previous decisions. Virtually every directive or other legal document will require your loved one's signature.

4. Take time with your loved one to discuss (and put in writing) what he or she wants at the end of life . . . a funeral, a celebration, buried in a casket, cremated, the remains placed in an urn and a columbarium, the ashes buried or sprinkled in a memorial garden, or whatever. Decide to which funeral home the loved one will be taken. It would even be well to discuss specific music, scripture passages, and the like for all services. Ideally, have the loved one help write the obituary. If necessary, do all of the above for yourself to keep from stressing out your loved one. This will be of great help to you and your children when you or your loved one dies. You will have limited time available later, so get it done early.

5. If you have family nearby, try to involve them as much as possible in the care of your loved one to keep you emotionally stable. If not, try to have close friends and your priest, minister, or deacon call or

visit you regularly to give you strength to deal with your emotional and faith journey. Our children lived far away so could not give me this support, and our pastors never visited. I had to rely mostly on friends from our church.

6. Remember to treat your loved one with affection and respect and focus on all the things he or she can do so you can enjoy as many years with each other as possible. Your loved one will become very sensitive to your moods and behavior, so your kindness, love, and even good humor become important in making your lives more enjoyable.

2

Second Year
of the Journey

JANUARY 2012 &

Dee and I resumed our normal active lives in Payson, but because of Dee's increasing insecurity and desire to have me nearby, I took yoga classes with her and she took art and crafts classes with me. Dee excelled in the yoga class, and even as a beginner she produced some nice acrylic paintings in the art class and a variety of interesting objects in the crafts class. She loved these activities. In early January we took two half-day ski trips with friends. Dee skied beautifully. We hoped and prayed that we could enjoy this activity for years to come.

The senior doctor at the Mayo Clinic called us the second week in January and asked if we could see him two weeks before our scheduled return visit. My hopes and fears multiplied. Did Dee have a disease that must be treated immediately? Did she have a tumor or something that must be removed? Why would the doctor call to have the appointment moved up unless it was urgent? We visited the doctor a long two weeks later with high hopes and fears.

Instead of announcing something dramatic, the doctor spent an hour going over the test results. Dee thought her memory had improved since the first neurological exam, but the tests showed that her memory and cognitive abilities had declined significantly. Her thyroid tested normal. There was no sign of mold in her system. Her blood count and all vital signs were normal. There was no sign of a brain tumor, blood clot, or any treatable condition in her brain. The doctor's prognosis was early-stage Alzheimer's disease, a mentally debilitating and progressive condition that might be slowed by treatment but for which there is no cure.

This news destroyed me. Dee did not appear to comprehend the significance of the prognosis, or at least hid her emotions. The doctor recommended that she continue to take Aricept, get plenty of exercise and rest, and to eat healthily. He advised us to focus on what Dee can do, not on what she can't do. We heartily agreed. But he also stated emphatically, "Because of Dee's decreased ability to process information, she should discontinue driving and any other physical activity requiring quick and correct responses." Dee did not like this advice. She would not give up driving.

In late January Dee's resolve changed. She drove home after a meeting at our church visibly shaken. When she showed me damage to the front fender and bumper of our pickup truck I asked her, "What did you hit?"

"A wall at the church," she replied.

She could not describe the wall, so I drove her to the church in our car and discovered that she had driven over a bumper in the parking lot, then swerved into an exterior wall of the men's restroom. She must have pressed on the gas pedal instead of the brake and could not think fast enough to change.

Dee decided then and there that she would no longer drive. I liked this decision a lot because she could have been hurt, or hurt someone else in another accident. And she likely would have been very stubborn if I had suggested that she quit driving. I enthusiastically supported her decision and repeatedly assured her of its wisdom. Happily, she did not change her mind. But of course this made me the sole driver on all trips and to all activities.

I told the chair of the trustees about the accident and arranged for our insurance company to pay for damages to the truck and building. The chair kept quiet about who ran into the church. This pleased us because we could keep Dee's memory problems to ourselves.

FEBRUARY–MARCH 2012 ৵

In February we decided to visit our oldest son and his family in New Mexico, but to break up the trip by skiing at our favorite ski area in eastern Arizona. We skied for nearly two days with no problems, but late on the second day Dee fell on an intermediate run near the top of the mountain. I helped her up and reminded her to lean forward if she hit an icy spot. However, near the bottom of the run, Dee hit another icy spot and pulled back. This time she fell hard on her bottom. I could tell by her screams that this hurt her badly, so I comforted her and did not try to get her up, fearing that she had broken something. The ski patrol came and took her to their shack, where she seemed to recover quickly. We then continued to drive on to New Mexico.

Dee indicated while we drove that her hip hurt a lot, so I pulled into a walk-in medical clinic in a small town near the eastern border of Arizona. The doctor on duty examined her and advised us to return as quickly as possible to the hospital in Show Low because he believed that she had fractured her pelvis. He said that if the fracture is bleeding Dee must have immediate treatment or the complications could be severe. So we drove back to the hospital, where they discovered a hairline fracture—not bleeding. However, they recommended that we return home immediately so Dee could get weight off her pelvis. We called our son and told him the unfortunate news. Dee followed directions and recovered quickly, but we agreed that she should not ski again.

We avoided physical activities throughout the winter but stayed active in the church. We sang in the choir and participated in a small group called Tables for Many. Dee did her best in every activity but increasingly lost her ability to communicate or follow directions. Most church members now recognized Dee's diminishing capabilities and did their best to assist her.

I began to attend an Alzheimer's support group in Payson that featured speakers with knowledge about how to deal with the disease and allowed members to discuss how to cope with it. I heard what seemed like horror stories about the behavior of some loved ones with Alzheimer's and felt fortunate because Dee remained the wonderful, loving person that I married over fifty years earlier. I could not imagine her otherwise and expressed this to the group. Several responded sadly, "Yes, my spouse [or parent] was like that during the early stages."

APRIL–AUGUST 2012 ❧

We began returning to New Mexico on a regular basis so I could arrange for subcontractors to complete construction of our cabin near our son's home. Dee enjoyed these trips. She never complained about anything. She liked driving across country and seeing sights along the way. She loved visiting our son, his wife, and our grandchildren. I did too, but I spent many hours arranging for subcontractors to accomplish their work.

Dee and I returned for a week in June and two weeks in early July to finish some interior work on the cabin. Our youngest son and his family came to New Mexico on the fourth of July so our whole family could be together for a few days. Dee beamed with joy with all of our family together, and no one seemed to notice (or at least no one commented about) Dee's memory loss.

SEPTEMBER–DECEMBER 2012 ❧

Dee and I returned to New Mexico several times to try to finish the cabin. My son and his boys helped me work on the interior. She mostly watched as we worked. We returned to the cabin for Christmas with bedding and some kitchen supplies so we could camp in the cabin while applying finishing touches. Dee really enjoyed these visits.

While Dee's Alzheimer's became apparent in the fall of 2010 with her forgetting a few proper nouns and having difficulty balancing the checkbook, now she cannot remember many proper nouns. She has a hard time remembering the day of the week, the time of day, and the names of people, even her grandchildren. This frustrates both of us because remembering names had been one of her strengths. Dee often forgets where she put something. She rarely remembers to close a door behind her, even the refrigerator door. She has a similar problem with flushing the toilet.

At times Dee becomes distraught about a missing object. I try to assure her that the object did not leave the house, so we go hunting until we find it ... where she left it. One day she could not find the scissors that she used to cut food products. They were nowhere to be found. We eventually found them, along with two rolls of plastic tape, in the birthday gift wrapping cabinet. "See," she said, "I told you. We always find them." I just grinned.

I now know that my primary responsibility is to show Dee that I love her and will not leave her. She really worries about this. She has said more than once that we should divorce so I can live a normal life. I usually reply, "It really hurts when you suggest divorce." This generally satisfies her. But if I am grumpy for any reason, Dee attributes my problem to her.

Dee and I need to express our love for each other, just as we have throughout our entire married lives. Loving activities are an important way for me to show her how much I love her. She is so insecure and dependent that having a satisfactory love life gives her a needed confidence boost.

Reflections on the Second Year ❧

Realizing that Dee had Alzheimer's disease and would not recover put me into an entirely different mindset. I read everything I could about the disease and how to deal with it. I joined a support group and began to get our affairs in order, including wills and other directives. I needed to do this while Dee could still agree to something and, especially, sign her name on documents. I dropped everything else to care for Dee and make arrangements for our future.

I felt trapped with the unfinished cabin in New Mexico and resolved to get it done quickly so that we could either move there near our son and his family or, alternatively, get rid of the old double-wide on the property and rent out the cabin. I also knew that our plans to travel to the East Coast and especially to South America were no longer possible. We had to begin living within Dee's diminishing capabilities. There were so many things I still wanted to do, and even some that Dee wanted to do, that were no longer feasible.

We had been so busy enjoying our retirement that we had not given a lot of thought to our own mortality. We expected to live for many years together . . . like forever. I even imagined natural death in each other's arms. So now came all the hard work to prepare for Dee's certain decline and death, and she did not have the mental or emotional capacity to help.

We liked our independence. Dee even made it clear that she did not want to move to the isolated cabin in the mountains east of Albuquerque. She wanted to stay in familiar Payson with all of her church friends. I now realize that it would have been better if we had moved earlier to live near our children during our retirement years. Too late! We now had to face the future without everyday family support.

Advice to Caregivers ॐ

1. Give thought to where you live, especially where you will live during retirement, in case a debilitating disease or injury should afflict you or your loved one. It is important to have family near to assist you and provide respite care.

2. Read everything you can about Alzheimer's disease and attend Alzheimer's Association conferences in your area to learn from knowledgeable persons what to do as the disease progresses. The time may come, as it did with me, when you cannot leave your loved one even to attend these events to obtain the information you desperately need.

3. Find and attend an Alzheimer's caregiver support group to learn about what may come next and how to cope with changes. The group members will listen, understand, and provide emotional support.

4. Develop a network of friends to support you emotionally. Friends from your place of worship or other organizations may provide the support you need during this early stage of the disease.

5. If you want people to remember your loved one as a once capable person, try to discover everything about his or her life before you met so you can tell your friends, children, and grandchildren.

6. Start lining up relatives and close friends to come to your home to provide you with some respite. Start this early so your loved one gets used to having them around and welcomes them as the disease progresses. You will need this support to accomplish household tasks and get away for a needed breather. You have no idea how much you will be stressed when caregiving becomes a 24/7 activity, or *The 36-Hour Day*, as that book describes it.

7. Driving is both the symbol and reality of independence for a person with Alzheimer's. I was fortunate that my wife had enough sense to give up driving after a minor accident in which no one was injured. However, do not be the one to insist that your loved one give up driving. You need to retain his or her trust. A family doctor or other respected person should make the case, or you may have to ask the motor vehicle department to take away your loved one's driver's license. Otherwise, an accident with injuries is a very distinct possibility because of the person's inability to think quickly and respond correctly.

8. Enjoy the good life with your loved one as long and as much as you can during this early stage of Alzheimer's. It may not last much longer.

3

Third Year
of the Journey

❧

In early January we told the Mayo Clinic doctor what had happened during the previous year. He said to keep up what we were doing and added a prescription for Namenda, a drug similar to Aricept that is supposed to improve memory and the ability to do daily activities.

We traveled to New Mexico several times to see our oldest son's family and arrange for subcontractors to install countertops and appliances in the cabin. I timed stops along the way to avoid urinary events in the vehicle and drank coffee to stay awake on the 350-mile journey.

Dee still does well in social settings and maintains close relationships with a number of women in our church. However, much like a child, she greets friends with excited hugs, kisses, and other expressions of her love. Her women friends reciprocate and do their best to make Dee feel comfortable. She understands some of what people say but cannot contribute her own thoughts. It frustrates her, but she generally remains positive.

The evening of April 30 marked a turning point in Dee's ability. She seemed confused and needed direction in every effort. She also expressed foreboding about the future. "Something very bad happening," she said. But she could not articulate what it was and lost her usual bright-eyed, cheerful, smiling disposition. This change was hard on both of us. After a good night's sleep on her part, not on mine, Dee awoke without this sense of foreboding. I felt a lot better with her happy again.

Showering together is the norm now because Dee cannot figure out how to get the water at the right temperature. She forgets to get the washcloths and towels ready before entering the shower and cannot remember how to wash her face or body. I undress and enter the shower to help her and finish my shower after getting her dry and dressed. She no longer can figure out what to wear or how to put on clothes. But she remains positive and enjoys having me help.

Dee has lost the ability to do anything requiring memory . . . pouring water from a pitcher, scrambling eggs or cooking anything, sewing on a button. I try to redirect and help her with a simpler task so she will not become too frustrated. She reads a lot but comprehends and remembers little. I am glad she tries. It must be good for her brain. She reads beside me in our office and frequently asks about the meaning of simple words that she no longer remembers.

Dee seldom remembers anything for even a few seconds. She calls for me to come quickly but when I arrive has no idea why she called. This frustrates her and stresses me. She forgets whether to put food products in the refrigerator or pantry, so she puts them in an empty space. Then she becomes upset when she cannot find them. So do I. She does not recognize named objects because she cannot remember what they look like. Occasionally she lashes out at me for not helping. She forgets to turn off lights and to flush the toilet. For Dee, out of sight is out of mind.

In spite of all this, Dee continues to be a loving person. Her faith in God does not waver. She is beautiful in her appearance and personality.

We share pleasant moments focusing on things she can do. She has good muscle memory and hits and putts golf balls pretty well. She also does well playing tennis, dancing, and bowling. This part of her brain function is thus far not impaired.

We do nearly everything together because Dee cannot stand it without me nearby. We take yoga, go to the gym, and enjoy art and crafts classes together. She produces some beautiful paintings, even as a beginner. She participates in social settings as an active listener but struggles to introduce a new thought. I try to help with words and she seems to appreciate my efforts.

One of Dee's amusing traits is her use of plural pronouns rather than singular. She refers to me as "the other people" in the house, "you guys," or "all of you." Less amusing is her use of the word "shit" when she is upset or startled. Indeed, it feels like I am raising a child in reverse.

We had a rare beam of hope when Dee's best friend received a stem cell infusion in Florida. Her lungs regenerated so much that her primary care doctor took her off hospice care. The doctor also claimed considerable success using stem cells for patients with Alzheimer's disease. I hoped this was true because it would be a lifesaver for Dee. I conducted an Internet search for testimonies from persons receiving the treatment and found none. Why not? If a person had been healed, wouldn't they want the world to know? But in the same sense, if the person had not been cured, wouldn't the caregiver who spent $32,500 want the world to know?

A similar facility on the West Coast does stem cell implants in Tijuana, Mexico. The doctors make claims and other doctors and writers make counterclaims about successes and failures, but their patients are silent. Another medical organization claims to have testimonials from patients. However, this organization will not reveal the testimonials because of doctor/patient privacy concerns. A different doctor wrote a book about how she cured her husband of Alzheimer's using coconut oil. I tried this product for several weeks with Dee and observed no beneficial effect. After considerable research, I decided not to consider stem cell implants or coconut oil as possible cures for Alzheimer's. The evidence convinced me that these treatments do not cure or halt the progression of this terrible disease. I believe they are scams.

We returned to the New Mexico cabin in early June with a U-Haul trailer full of furnishings so that we could use the unfinished cabin as a second home. I say "we" meaning that I worked on the cabin and Dee watched. She tried to help but couldn't understand directions. She occasionally handed me tools and helped clean up. I mostly tried to keep her in a safe place to watch. We also selected a real estate agent to sell the vacant double-wide on the property.

Dee is now losing long-term memory. She is forgetting almost everything about her past. I try to help by going over picture albums and memory books with her. She does not recognize many objects around the house. If I ask her to turn on a light, she looks around, even at the light switch, and does not recognize it. My heart aches to see her life passing in this dreadful way.

The most frustrating part of my day is trying to get Dee clean before going to bed. She runs out of steam in early evening, gets upset, and resists doing almost anything, including eating her dinner. She just wants to go to bed without washing up or even getting into her pajamas. I do my best to get her to brush her teeth and wash her face. But it does not always work. I have to help her wash her face, make sure she brushes and flosses her teeth, and help her put on pajamas, all over her very strong objections and resistance. She will not wear adult diapers at night even though she cannot get up quickly enough to avoid wetting her pajamas and the sheets.

Sundowning, as described in the Alzheimer's research literature, is real. If you need to do something with a loved one with Alzheimer's, it is best to do it in the morning, or at the latest in the early afternoon. You are in for a difficult time in the late afternoon and early evening.

We returned to New Mexico early in July, after buyers removed the double-wide from the site, and enjoyed spending time with our son and his family. However, Dee urinated while sitting in a Sunday school class.

Our son, sitting next to her, heard the urine dripping through the perforated plastic chair seat but thoughtfully waited until after the class to clean up while I took Dee to the men's bathroom to change her into dry panties and slacks.

A few days later we visited a shut-in friend in Payson, where Dee wet her pants while waiting for the man to open the front door. Dee also farted loudly three times in company the following day and apparently did not realize it. Several people in the Alzheimer's support group recounted similar embarrassing actions by their loved one, so I resigned myself to more of the same.

AUGUST–SEPTEMBER 2013 ❧

Dee agreed to wear adult diapers on a trip to New Mexico to house-sit for our son's family while they went on vacation, but on the morning of our departure she would not wear them. Indeed, she hid the box of diapers. After she screamed at me several times, I said, "Okay, let's give it another try," and took along extra clothes, expecting that she would soil them. We had to change her clothes twice on the way to New Mexico. Urinary incontinence is now usual.

After our son's family left on their vacation, I rented a small bulldozer to grade the earth where the double-wide had been to create a place to park cars near the entry door to the cabin. I then used the dozer to place asphalt millings stored on the site as a parking surface. I could not let Dee come outside with me because I could easily run over and severely injure or kill her. So I made her stay in the cabin or on the decks to watch me. She hated this! She hated me! She hated the cabin! She fretted, cried, and threatened to kill herself. She also stormed out of the cabin and walked down the road toward our son's house several times. A few times she went the other way onto undeveloped land north of the cabin. Thankfully, she usually turned around and I found her coming back.

It was no fun for her or me, but I felt that I had to get this final bit of work done so we could rent out the cabin to help cover the increasing costs for her care in Payson. I finished the work in five days and then gave my full attention to Dee. Too late! She was not doing well. Her anger with me was palpable and her willingness to do anything had vanished.

OCTOBER 2013 ॐ

On October 5 I awakened to discover that Dee had defecated in her pajamas and made a mess on the way to the bathroom. I cleaned her and the messes in the bed and on the floor. I also convinced her to put on a diaper, tucked her into my bed, and stayed up to put all the soiled items in the washer and write this story.

I prayed constantly for a miracle. I had more than the "faith of a mustard seed," believing that God would intervene and restore Dee to full health. She had always been the rock of faith in our marriage and lived it every day in her thoughts, prayers, and actions. She treated her body as a temple, never abusing it in any way. She did everything she could to protect herself from Alzheimer's disease, but she got it anyway. And my prayers have not been answered.

I ask, would a loving God want Dee to slip into this world of unknowing? Could this serve God's purpose or plan in some way? I cannot imagine how. My conclusion is that God no longer performs miracles like those described in the New Testament. Maybe by praying we receive the wherewithal to cope with our problems, but this is small comfort to a guy losing his wife day by day. It breaks my heart to see Dee struggle. She's losing the battle. She knows it and I know it.

As one friend whose mother died of Alzheimer's told me, it is the long goodbye. I hate it! I am angry with God! More than ever I wonder if God exists. Is our condition simply a matter of evolution that will last until the weaker are weeded out and only the strong remain?

Once we planned to grow old in the home I designed for us in Payson and to enjoy lots of good times with our friends, children, and grandchildren. Dee loves this house, loves living here, loves her friends, and loves the neighborhood. So do I. I continue to love her very much and want to help her remain positive. Now I envision a time when I cannot care for her.

A few minutes alone apparently seems like forever to Dee. If I go downstairs, even after telling her where I am going, she gets upset and wanders around the house looking for me. We now go around the house together, sit at the computer together, watch TV together, read together, and grocery shop together so she will not feel abandoned. It terrifies her not to be with me or with someone she knows and loves. She is no longer the brilliant leader, organizer, and speaker who never doubted her abilities and traveled by herself all over the country to get her education and accomplish her professional work. She could do anything she set out to do. No more.

Something humorous, at least to others, now happens. When Dee answers the phone, she says, "Hello," very sweetly. When the person responds, Dee repeats what she heard. If they ask for me, Dee puts down the phone and looks for me, but forgets why. The person on the phone is left hanging while Dee wanders around the house. I eventually find a phone off the hook and replace it. Dee, of course, has no memory of who tried to contact me or even that they called.

One evening late in October the fireworks began at bedtime. Dee did not understand why she should take any pills and screamed at me something about God. Ear piercing!

"Just take the pills and get it over with!" I yelled back.

"Why?!"

"They are for Alzheimer's disease."

"I am not sick!" she screamed in response.

"Please take the pills so we can go to bed," I implored.

She put one pill in her mouth but would not swallow it. Then she pushed the glass of water away and screamed as loud as she could. I slapped her on her fanny like I did with the boys during their terrible twos and told her to calm down. To my surprise, Dee clenched her fists and began swinging at me, hitting me a couple of times on my chest. This must have hurt her wrists or fists because she quit swinging, washed down the pill in her mouth, and took the other pills.

I told her to go to bed and did not tuck her in or kiss her good night. I felt totally disrespected and could not control my anger, even knowing objectively that Dee was not herself. Because she had no short-term memory, the whole episode vanished for her and she went right to sleep. However, it upset me so much that I could not sleep. I tossed and turned, wondering why God allows people to get this terrible disease, particularly people like Dee who have been constant in their faith and dedicated to the work of the church. I received no answer.

I also wonder why Dee should take any pills. They only prolong her (and my) misery. They certainly are not curing her and don't even claim to. I called the doctor's nurse about this and she said she would talk to the doctor. At this writing I have no answer from the doctor.

On a Tuesday in mid-October, a very thoughtful lady from our church arranged for two ladies to take Dee to a movie and have ice cream afterward. With Dee gone, I cleaned my desk and did the books while a tech worked on my computer. Dee was happy when she returned, but not happy to see the tech. She screamed at him to go home and badgered him until he did. She watched me for a while after he left as I tried to catch up on three weeks of emails, but then she began to throw my papers into the wastebasket. I became very upset as I dug through the trash looking for missing papers. I scolded her loudly and she hit me hard on the back with both fists. I became very angry and shouted, "Get out of here and stay away from me!" She left but came back later to apologize and say that she wouldn't bother me again. I certainly hoped so but had my doubts given her lack of memory.

I awoke in the middle of the night with a bad case of heartburn and ended up taking several antacid and anti-gas pills. I tried to sleep by resting on my knees while leaning over a hot pad on the bed but with little success. I could not believe this was really happening. It was a nightmare.

Late in October we reached another sobering turning point. I tried to give Dee a hug when I returned from the men's Bible study but she pushed me away and angrily asked, "Who are you?"

Startled, I replied, "I'm your husband! We've been married for over fifty-two years and have two sons."

She seemed surprised, calmed down, and asked about our boys. I told her about our sons and about their wives and our grandchildren. She had forgotten. I knew this would happen someday, but I was not ready for it.

Dee willingly showers with me on Sunday mornings and loves putting on her nice Sunday clothes, earrings, and the like. She still puts on a little eye shadow and lipstick and looks really good both to herself and to me. Then she loves to greet everyone at church as if she were still an active ordained deacon. For her, church is the best place, the safest place. Her life and mine would be so much better if Sundays happened every day of the week.

NOVEMBER 2013 ❧

Dee's best friend from Kansas and her husband visited us early in the month, arriving shortly after we finished lunch. Dee gave the man a brief hug, but she and the woman hugged and held onto each other for several minutes. The woman is in the early stages of dementia and showing symptoms similar to Dee's in 2010. After I put Dee to bed, the couple and I exchanged stories about what is happening in our lives.

The next two days with our friends went well, but Dee became upset when the husband and I left to attend the men's Bible study breakfast on Wednesday morning. Dee was so upset that her friend called her husband during the breakfast and talked with him to calm herself. She told him that Dee wanted to live with them in Missouri. I told him that Dee had already asked her elderly aunt in Colorado to take care of her. The aunt told Dee that it would be best to stay with me.

Dee and I saw a new neurologist in Payson a week later. She was kind and gentle as she tried to determine Dee's capabilities. She supports what I am trying to do and suggested that we take Dee off Namenda for six weeks to see if it contributes to her rapid mood swings from love, to anger, to occasional violence against me. I welcomed this trial.

Dee angrily yelled at me the next day when dressing after a yoga class, "I have no clothes to wear!"

"You have lots of clothes in your three closets. Levi's and a blouse should work today," I told her.

"I have neither! You have everything, all the money and all the clothes!" she shouted.

I took out all six pairs of her Levi's and placed them on the bed for her to see. She jerked the black pair off the bed and shouted, "I have no blouse!"

I showed her dozens of blouses in her closet and told her, "Pick one and quit bellyaching."

"You are a really bad man!" she screamed.

This hurt and made me angry so I screamed back, "Just dress yourself!" and left the room. I've been angry all day. I know it is the disease, but I have feelings too and they are badly damaged.

I eventually helped Dee put on her clothes, but lunch was no pleasure with both of us still angry. Another lady friend who helps us with housework came in the early afternoon to take Dee out, but Dee remained in a very dark mood and tried to jump out of the moving pickup truck at the main intersection in town. I apologized to the lady for Dee's conduct and for not telling her about our morning conflict. I had hoped that Dee would like getting away from the "really bad man." Obviously, something is going on with Dee that I do not understand.

While they were gone for about two hours, I vacuumed all of the carpets and hard surface floors and scrubbed the kitchen and bathroom floors. I swept pine needles off the driveway and sidewalks and filled the trash can for pick up the next day. I worked like mad . . . because I was mad and everything needed to be done. Nothing improved my mood.

Dee and I watched TV that evening for a while but she got up repeatedly to wander down the hall. I followed her to make sure she did not destroy something important. Dee went to the bedroom soon after seven and to my amazement took off her clothes, put on pajamas, pulled back her covers, and got in bed all by herself. I turned off the lights and came into the office to write about another day in the life of the Alzheimer's patient and caregiver.

When we got up the next Sunday, Dee felt very low and refused to wash or exercise. "Going to die today," she said. Then she asked me, "Please help me die."

"Sweetheart, I can't help you die. I'll end up in jail!" I replied.

Nevertheless, she persisted with her intent to die and tore the sheets and blankets off the twin beds.

"It won't look good with the sheets off the beds if you die today," I told her. "You might want the house to look better." This seemed to ring a bell in her head and she helped me remake the beds.

When we finished I said, "It will look better if you are clean and nicely dressed when you die. We should take the shower I suggested earlier."

She agreed. So we selected clothes for her to wear, put them on the bed, and took a shower together. Fortunately, she quickly forgot her earlier death wish. Then we ate breakfast, read the funnies, and went to church.

She seemed quite happy and sure of herself in church, even greeting a number of people several times before and after the service. After the service she invited a few friends to go to lunch with us. Some accepted and we had a nice lunch at a small restaurant in town.

After lunch Dee and I agreed to take a walk to visit a friend in a nearby health care facility. After visiting with him for a while Dee said, "We must go home now." We said goodbye and started to walk home.

Along the way Dee said, "I never want to live in one of those places." I reassured her that I would do everything I could to keep her with me at home. "I don't want to live with you, either," she told me.

She maintained that position when we arrived home, saying, "You are a very bad man. I'm leaving." She then stormed out the front door, but once outside and sensing the cold, she came back in and said emphatically, "I am hungry!" I quickly heated up some chicken noodle soup. She helped a little by cutting some goat cheese to put in the soup and then ate her soup and some crackers.

Dee calmed down after she ate, and I tried to explain what the Alzheimer's was doing to her. I emphasized that her bad behavior results from the disease. I also told her, "You are my sweetheart and I love you very much." She seemed happy enough with the discussion and my expression of love for her. After dinner she took her two pills and we headed for bed. I hope she wakes up refreshed and we have a couple more good days together.

We experienced more of the same for the rest of the month—some good times but mostly bad. Dee often hid or misplaced various objects and then beat on me until I pinned her down. She acted as if possessed by a demon. Then she would say, "I want to live with [someone's name]," and I would respond, "Go ahead. Find someone who wants to live with a person who beats on them. Good luck."

The neurologist suggested, and I agreed, that Dee should visit her primary care doctor to see if a urinary tract infection was causing her recent bad behavior. If tests prove negative then the neurologist will consider something to calm Dee.

DECEMBER 2013 ❧

One morning Dee ripped off my suspenders, threw them on the floor, and once again shouted, "You have all the clothes and I have nothing!" I showed her the clothes in her closets and dresser drawers, but she returned to my closet and started throwing suspenders and shirts on the floor. I grabbed one of her arms and she swung at me with the other. So I grabbed both arms, pushed her back into the bedroom, and pinned her to the bed. She quaked with anger but finally relaxed and said, "You always win." Indeed! I don't feel like a winner. My life is a mess.

Another morning after a phone call I told Dee, "The lady who arranges for other ladies to visit and go to the movies with you wants to take you to breakfast. It would be nice if you were clean for the day's activities." Dee would not cooperate, so I called the lady and suggested that she might not want to come, but she insisted. So I agreed reluctantly and told Dee that her friend would arrive soon. Dee then wanted to take the shower. When the lady arrived early, Dee ran out of the shower, nude and half dry, into the lady's arms, pleading with her to take her away from "this man."

I finished drying and slipped on my bathrobe as the lady helped Dee into her clothes. They then went out for breakfast and to the church to pack bags of food for homeless kids. Dee panicked when they got to the church, fearing that "the man" would be there, and refused to get out of the car. So the lady took Dee to her home and called to let me know. I thanked her profusely and asked if Dee could stay with her overnight and for breakfast. She agreed to this.

When I called in the morning, the lady said, "Dee is still afraid of 'the man' and is having rapid mood swings." We agreed that it would be better for Dee to stay with her through lunch, both of us hoping that a good meal would calm her and she would forget about "the man." We also agreed to have the lady bring Dee to the doctor's office to check for the suspected urinary tract infection.

I got to the doctor's office before they did and told the nurse what had happened. I showed her pictures of my bruises and abrasions from Dee's flailing away at me the previous few days and asked her to check to see if Dee had any bruises from my grabbing and lifting her by the arms. I had not seen any but wanted the nurse to check because I did not want to be accused of battering my sick wife.

When the lady, her husband, and Dee arrived at the doctor's office, Dee recognized and sat next to me on the couch, much to my surprise. The visit turned out well, with the lady helping Dee provide a urine sample and the doctor finding that Dee did, indeed, have a urinary tract infection. The lady and her husband, seeing that Dee now responded well to me, chose to leave her with me.

My God, I thought. *Dee's violent behavior is caused by a bladder infection and she has no way of letting me know.* I felt really bad about how I reacted to her violent attacks.

The next day, after twelve and a half hours of sleep, Dee refused to swallow the prescribed antibiotic. She held it in her mouth then spit it in her glass. I fished it out and gave it back to her, but she threw it on the floor. When I offered her a new pill, she threw it behind some dishes and said, "Just kill me!"

"Sweetheart, I don't want to kill you. I am trying to help you cure your bladder infection," I told her. Frustrated, I called our primary care doctor and the neurologist to find out what to do next.

The neurologist told me we must clear up the infection before giving Dee more drugs. Our primary care doctor's nurse said she could give Dee the antibiotic in one big shot. Wonderful! When we arrived at the doctor's office the nurse gave Dee the shot without any complaints.

By this time it really registered with me how much pain Dee must have endured with this urinary tract infection. She had not grabbed her tummy or expressed her pain in words. Going forward I will be more alert to symptoms.

It is so hard to lose the love of my life a little bit more each day with no prospect of improvement or cure. Can purgatory be any worse than this? I doubt it. No! We are there now.

The nurse called later in the week and said that by now Dee should be over her urinary tract infection and asked if her behavior had improved. "Not really," I responded. However, now that the antibiotic has gone through her system and Dee has not taken any pill in over a week, she is in a much better mood. We had two days of peace and most of the time she was very loving. This is a marvelous change. I hope it continues.

One morning Dee was very much into hugging and kissing and we made love for the first time in several months. She wanted to make love again in the early evening while we sat together on the living room couch watching the news on TV. We began to undress, but fears overcame her as we got into bed and she simply wanted to go to sleep. So I helped her into her pajamas, tucked her into bed and told her that I loved her, and gave her a tender goodnight kiss. I left the door ajar so she could see that I was in the office and she soon fell fast asleep.

Dee now screams "Hello!" even when I am next to her. I suggest that she simply ask, "Bob, where are you?" then I will say, "I'm not leaving you. I'll always be near." She apologizes and says that she will not shout or scream again. But she cannot remember.

On our walk today, when I was just a step in front of her, she suddenly screamed, "Where are you?!" She apparently looked back and did not see me. I feel so bad for her and yet can do nothing to improve her condition except to give her my love. I call it "love medicine." I think it is better than drugs.

Many words now mean practically nothing to Dee. She repeats words like table, drawer, place mat, or spoon without the least understanding of their meaning. I try to define or rephrase the words but this does not help. When I read her the funnies, with pictures as supporting information, she seems to understand and laughs heartily with me at times. She loves to sing with me at home and at church, where she seems to be in a very special comfort zone. She has a beautiful soprano voice and sings joyously in time and on key with the music, but the words are not there, just gibberish.

Dee picked up an envelope on the stair rail today with a check in it to a utility company and tore it in half. Thankfully she put the two halves back down on the rail. She means no harm and is apologetic, but she will do the same thing again if I leave out another envelope. To watch her can be humorous, fascinating, irritating, and heartbreaking all at the same time.

We are now receiving Christmas cards on a regular basis. Dee remembers only a few of the people who sent them. I try to help her remember by showing her their pictures and saying their names repeatedly. I am hoping that we are through the angry phase of Alzheimer's and Dee will return to her loving self. Getting rid of the urinary tract infection was key. Maybe not taking any medication is another key. Now I can show my love for Dee even as I would to a very small child and she can reciprocate with love for me as well. We do not need to make love, only to love and be loved. I can handle that.

Is it Dr. Jekyll or Mrs. Hyde? Or is Dee the little girl who could be very good or very bad and sometimes just horrible? Which will it be today? I never know. Dee started out the day as a loving wife but by late morning became agitated and mean while I spoke on the phone to a person about selling our land in New Mexico to help cover the increasing costs for Dee's care. Dee picked up papers off my desk and started taking them out of the room. I had to chase after her to retrieve them. She then took papers out of my New Mexico construction files. I had to grab them before she could hide or tear them up. Finally, I told the person on the line, "I have to discontinue the call because a very sick person is making it impossible for me to continue." Frustrating!

I straightened out the papers and files and left the room, hoping Dee would follow. She did, but when I tried to lock the door behind us, she began to hit me, stood in the doorway, and refused to budge. So I gave up and said, "I'm leaving." I headed for the front door with her following, begging me not to go and pledging to be good. I stayed, but by that time I was in no mood to accept her empty promises and had a splitting headache. Life now is so difficult.

One Wednesday in mid-December began much better when I told Dee that she would be going out for breakfast with her best friend. I asked her to get up right away so she could shower and get ready. The shower went well, with her washing her own hair and body without my help. We got to the restaurant just as the lady arrived, so I turned Dee over to her and went into the men's Bible study breakfast in an adjoining room. Dee's breakfast apparently went well, but with her looking into our room occasionally to make sure I had not left.

When we got home, I began to clean off some moldy caulk in the shower. Dee watched for a little while, then suddenly closed the glass door tight against the frame to trap me in the shower. I pleaded for her to let me out because it was hot in the enclosure with the floor heat on. She would not open the door and resisted when I tried to open it. I pulled so hard that the pull gave way and the door opened.

"Get out!" I commanded. "You're more trouble than you're worth."

Dee ran toward the front of the house but stopped in the kitchen and screamed, "Just kill me!"

"I can't!" I yelled back.

"I'll kill myself!" she screamed, and began to look for something to do it with. Fortunately, I now keep the knives and other possible weapons out of sight where she cannot find them. She cannot even remember how to open a drawer.

Once again Dee apologized. "I am sorry! I'll never cause you trouble again."

"Fine," I said, and headed to the master bathroom with her close behind. "Will you be good?" I asked. "If so, please sit on the blue recliner until I finish cutting off the old caulk."

Amazingly, she did. She sat there for quite a while and began to clean her fingernails. Then she called to me and asked if she could look at her jewelry. I told her yes and she spent the rest of the time sorting through jewelry and, I am sure, misplacing a number of pieces while I finished cleaning the shower. But at least she stayed out of my way until I came to the bedroom later and told her, "Lunch is ready."

The neurologist feels that there is no use trying to force Dee to take medications or food she does not want, but given Dee's violent behavior she recommended and prescribed a low dosage (25 mg) of quetiapine, an antipsychotic drug. It is supposed to work gradually to mellow Dee's behavior and can be made into powder and given to her with food. The pills are very small and Dee readily took one with water before dinner. I am hoping for the best.

After the neurology appointment we visited a friend at a local health care facility, where I talked with the admissions officer about what might happen if I get injured or sick and cannot care for Dee. She said that they have appropriate facilities to care for Dee. They just need a doctor's order.

Until Dee got Alzheimer's we thought we were bulletproof, so we had not acquired long-term care insurance. Now I am considering options for Dee's care if I am unable to care for her. Along that line, late this past September I contacted an attorney specializing in applications for the Arizona Long Term Care System (ALTCS), a version of Medicaid, because our savings are depleting. I came away with the impression that Dee would not qualify, that she was not far enough along with the disease to make a credible application. I think it is time to contact him again.

This is now becoming like a daily diary because everything is changing so fast. What started as an entry every few months, then weekly, has become an almost daily recount that I type after Dee is in bed asleep so I can unload the day in order to get some sleep.

FRIDAY, DECEMBER 20, 2013 ❧

Dee would not get up after thirteen hours in bed yesterday so I began to do things around the house. At fourteen hours I finally woke her up, but she immediately said, "I am not getting up. I'm going to die."

"Maybe, but it's up to God to decide if you're ready," I responded.

Nevertheless, Dee repeated that she would die, even after I reminded her of our plans to see a good friend in Phoenix.

"I don't want to see her," Dee said, then pleaded, "Kill me. Please kill me."

"I'm so sorry," I said. "I can't do it. It's against the law." I let her stay in bed and left the room.

I then checked the small print about the new pill. It clearly stated that if given to a person with dementia it might cause depression, thoughts of suicide, or even death. *Good grief*, I thought. *Don't doctors ever read the side effects of the medications they prescribe?*

I called the neurologist's office and left a message expressing my concern that the pill has the opposite effect from what it claims. The doctor's nurse called back after several of my calls and messages and said, "The doctor says to take Dee to the emergency room if you think she is in serious trouble."

This reflects poorly on the professionalism of the doctor, I thought.

Dee became agitated on the way to Phoenix, kicked the dashboard several times, hit her side door hard with her hands, and tried to open the door to get out. I pulled her back and pleaded with her to be good. But she was confused and angry while asking me questions about her father, brother, and mother. When I told her that they had all passed away, she became furious and blamed me for not letting her know. This went on and on until she decided she wanted to go home immediately. "I can't turn around in the middle of a divided highway," I told her. This made her madder and she kicked and hit whatever she could, including me. I begged her to be nice and shouted, "I can't drive while being hit!" She relented and pledged to be good but insisted that we go home as soon as I could turn around. I reminded her that her good friend planned to treat us to a Christmas dinner at the fancy Mansion Club next to the Biltmore Hotel.

When we arrived at the club Dee seemed happy to see and dine with her friend. Dee and I ordered salmon as the main course, butternut squash as a side, and an asparagus salad to start. When the salad came, even before the first taste, Dee proclaimed loudly, "I don't like it." She then complained at full volume about the squash. Her friend, not having seen

Dee for several months, quickly realized how her condition had deteriorated, especially when she picked up the salmon steak with her hands.

"Can I cut your salmon into small pieces so you can eat with your fork?" I asked. Dee nodded affirmatively. However, as is usual now, I had to remind her how to eat, to keep the napkin on her lap, to hold food over her plate, to lean forward, and so on. Her friend was clearly astonished by Dee's diminished capacity to think and do things. I told her that Dee had been voted Most Sophisticated in her senior class in high school. Clearly this is no longer the case.

When we got to the motel Dee said she would not go in. So, exasperated once again, I said, "Fine! I'll go in and you can sleep in the car." However, when I began to leave, Dee called for me to help and I returned to loosen her seat belt. She was not happy but came along. However, when we got to the room she hit me hard twice in the ribs before I could put down the suitcase to defend myself. "That hurts!" I cried out, and pleaded with her to be good. Again she looked really sorry and asked me to forgive her, saying she would not do it again. "I forgive you, Sweetheart!" I said.

But later, when I turned my back to her to brush my teeth, she hit me hard in the kidney area of my lower back. That really did hurt. She then declared, "I'm walking home."

"Go ahead, please!" I replied. But she could not figure out how to get out. And so it went until we finally had her pajamas on. But she would not go to bed until I did. By that time I was emotionally and physically exhausted and happy to comply. However, in my rush to leave that morning I forgot to pack my wedge pillow so I had to use the motel's four very hard overstuffed pillows to prop myself up. My stomach produced acid big time so that I could not lie flat on the bed. Clearly, this was one of the worst days of my life and probably Dee's as well. She soon fell asleep while I tried to get comfortable. It was not easy, so I got practically no sleep that night.

Dee thanked me for helping after her shower in the morning. She then said in her sweetest voice that she would like to go shopping. I called our friend and told her about Dee's desire to go shopping and agreed to meet her for lunch at the Phoenix Art Museum before attending a live performance of *White Christmas* at the adjacent theater. The friend asked how it went after we left her at the Biltmore. I said not so good and told her what happened. Dee listened but understood little of what I said so did not seem at all bothered. She was just happy to go shopping.

We went to Dillard's in Scottsdale, where I bought Dee two pairs of fine leather gloves and a beautiful plaid blouse. Dee was happy the whole time. However, on the way to the museum Dee asked why her brother was not with us. When I told her that he died several years earlier, she swung open the car door and thrust her body toward the door just as I made a left turn onto Twenty-Fourth Street from Camelback Road, both major streets with lots of traffic. Thankfully the seat belt stopped her until I could grab and hold her left arm while trying to maneuver through two busy lanes of traffic with my left hand to where I could stop and close the door. This was about as scary as anything you can imagine. We made it to the right lane in about two blocks, where I turned onto a side street and pulled the door shut. When I asked Dee to be nice and not spoil our day, she looked sorry and said she would try but soon asked why we could not go to see her aunt in Colorado. I tried to explain about the distance and then to distract her by talking about the fun we would have with our friend.

When we looked for our friend at the art museum, Dee shouted, "You're lying! She's not coming!" I insisted that the lady would arrive any moment, but Dee did not think so. When our friend came in, Dee ran to meet her, gave her a big hug, and all of Dee's worries vanished. We went into the restaurant and ordered sandwiches with sides of salad. Dee wanted what her friend ordered. So I ordered her a fruit salad and Diet Coke, but Dee could not understand why the salad and drink did not come immediately. A minute must seem like an eternity to her. When the salad and drink came, Dee ate and drank them right away. This made me happy because fruits and Coke contain lots of water. Yippee for hydration! Down with constipation (a current problem)! Happiness is relative. Really relative.

The *White Christmas* musical hit the spot with its fast-paced music, singing, and dancing. Dee clearly enjoyed the performance. She moved and sang along with the very good singers and dancers. When Bob sang *How much do I love you?* tears dripped down my cheeks as I thought about the wonderful love Dee and I had shared through many years and how much I miss it as Alzheimer's destroys her mind and personality. It is not right for this to happen to her and to our relationship. I am so often confronted with her negative behavior that I can hardly remember how wonderful, capable, and loving she once was.

On the way home, Dee could not recall anything about the play, even as I sang the songs to her. But she remained surprisingly calm and peaceful during our drive home and as we took our belongings upstairs and prepared for bed. She willingly brushed her teeth, flossed, and smiled as I tucked her into bed, gave her a big kiss, and said, "I love you, Sweetheart." She fell asleep almost immediately.

An hour later she called out for me and asked, "What are you doing?"

"I'm writing a story about the good times we had today with our friend," I replied. This seemed to satisfy her and she went back to sleep. Soon thereafter, however, she called for me to come. When I did, I found her on the toilet trying to wipe herself after a very big dump. Her backside was a mess and I was pleased to help her clean up. What a relief. The constipation was gone. I once took great pleasure in conversing, dancing, skiing, fly-fishing, traveling, and making love with Dee. Now I take pleasure in cleaning up her rear end. Amazing!

SUNDAY, DECEMBER 22, 2013 ๛

Dee once again refused to wake up after fourteen hours in bed. Finally she got up and rushed into the bathroom for a second large dump. This time I helped her clean up before she made a big mess. We brushed our teeth and hair and she put on her lipstick and jewelry after breakfast. She looked gorgeous as always and even smiled at herself in the mirror. We got to church just before eleven. All went well as she enjoyed visiting with her many friends before and after the service. We went out to lunch with some of these friends, but Dee spilled chili on her clothes and would eat no more. She ate only a bite of a chocolate chip cookie for dessert.

All in all, I would say we had a good day until Dee had diarrhea and soiled her pajamas and all of the bed sheets. I got her up and into the bathroom, dripping liquid poop all the way. Then she pooped all over the toilet and floor before landing on the toilet seat. She continued to have diarrhea for some time while I took off her pajamas and tried to clean up her bottom, legs, feet, the floor, and the toilet. Eventually it seemed as if she was finished, so I had her stand up to clean her more thoroughly by her sink. But as I finished she squirted out a whole lot more onto the floor and mirror and into a wicker wastebasket near the wall. I had her sit on the toilet again for a while and a lot more liquid poop came out. Finally, I got her cleaned up enough to put on a diaper that I found hidden behind the TV. I also remade the bed with three pads to keep the mattress clean should she have to go again. I tucked her back into bed, told her that I loved her, and began to clean up the mess in the bathroom. The stink was really bad so I got a plastic laundry basket and put the soiled linens, pajamas, rags, towels, and washcloths in it. I threw the wastebasket into the outside trash and put the soiled fabrics in the washer, set it on hot water and heavy duty, put in lots of soap, and hit the on button while holding my breath.

So we went from the frying pan into the fire. Undoubtedly, constipation was easier on me. And I am getting a much clearer picture of what mothers go through caring for sick children. It is a tough role: cook, housekeeper, maid, groundskeeper, maintenance person, nurse, caregiver. Hats off to the mothers of the world! And now I am one, at least in what I do. The whole thing would be a bit comical if it weren't happening to me.

MONDAY, DECEMBER 23–WEDNESDAY, DECEMBER 25, 2013 ❧

The following is from an email I sent to our sons on the twenty-third:

[Sons],

Dee and I had a pretty good day yesterday until about 10 p.m. when she woke up with diarrhea and made a mess all over the bathroom and again when I had begun to clean her at the sink. I re-made the bed and cleaned up Dee and the floor, wall, and trash can and had her back in bed by about 11:00 p.m. Then at about 11:30 p.m. she awoke again while I was cleaning the bathroom counter and barfed several times in the sink . . . most of it hitting accurately. This clogged up the sink, so I had to wait until about 12:30 a.m. to clean it and the stopper. I got to bed at about 1 a.m. after giving Dee a drink of water. She woke up about every hour thereafter needing a drink, so my sleep was limited during the night. We did not get up until 10 this morning. Dee drank a full glass of water and participated as best she could in our yoga exercises. She seemed to be feeling quite fit and completely finished with her upset stomach so I fixed our usual cereal and juice breakfast but Dee would not eat. At about 11 a.m. she indicated that she was hungry and agreed to eat toast and scrambled eggs. But she would have none of either after I made them. She did drink some water. A lady friend is picking her up in a few minutes. Maybe she can get Dee to eat something.

I am also concerned about the safety of driving the 6 hours to ABQ because of the possibility of more diarrhea and Dee's frequent mood changes. She has been hallucinating all morning as she looks at family pictures and wonders why we can't just stop everything and go visit everyone. She really does not get it that her mother, father and brother as well as my parents have passed on. She says right now (sitting next to me) that she will be good all of the way to ABQ, but who knows? Alzheimer's does strange things to her. My confidence in the neurologist is shaken, but I will call the family doctor to see if he thinks there is something I can give Dee that will help.

Relative to incontinence, Dee wore adult diapers and did not object to the mattress pads for the first time in months last night after the diarrhea episode. She would not wear adult diapers today, but promises (as she has before) that she will wear them on the trip. Here again what she promises today may not be what she does tomorrow or when she is at your home. I have the adult diapers and can bring them, but do not count on her wearing them.

I know that Dee and I would like to come and visit for Christmas, but I cannot predict anything about her behavior along the way or at your home. Quite frankly I am exhausted both physically and emotionally and doubt I would do well on the long trip. I will be cleaning the house and finish washing and drying the clothes now that Dee (just picked up) is with her lady friend. It's hard to get anything done around here when she is with me.

I would appreciate your advice given what I have just told you.

Love,

Dad

The following is from my youngest son to me and copied to his brother:

Dad,

I'm so, so sorry to hear all this bad news about Mom and the emotional and physical stress that you are experiencing right now. The main things I want you to know, Dad, is that we all love you and Mom so very much. Dad, you are doing such a FANTASTIC job in a truly difficult situation. You are a model Dad, even in the depths of this stressful, stressful time. I have always been exceedingly proud to be your son, but never more than now. I am so impressed by how well you are handling all this stuff (for lack of a better word). I also know that everyone, including you, has limits to how much they can do in certain situations. And I think we're now reaching the limit of even your incredible abilities. Thus, I think we need to get you more significant help right away to care for Mom, and to protect your own health and well-being. And, while I know trying to maintain some semblance of a normal life with social outings might seem like a good thing for your sanity, I would encourage you to minimize long-distance travels and outings that, I suspect, are only going to add to your stress.

I so wish that the first drug prescribed for Mom's frustrating, and even dangerous, behaviors would have worked miracles. It may be that we need to try that same drug again for a longer period of time, to let Mom's body adjust to it. Or, it may be that we need a totally different and perhaps more powerful drug that (sad as it may sound) just keeps her calm instead of driving you completely crazy with her happiness one minute and then hitting you hard the next minute, etc. Obviously, I'm no expert on the disease or the treatment options, but something else clearly needs to be done. Moreover, I believe it's true that, if we could go back in time and ask Mom what she would want us to do in this situation, she would be horrified by the thought of her hitting you and making you crazy, and maybe even injuring you, in this way. I, certainly, would want to be drugged, rather than hit anyone I loved so much even once, much less repeatedly. I can't imagine Mom saying anything different when she was of sound mind.

Of course, I so wish everything were different for you both, with just "normal" aging issues. But, we don't have that luxury here, so I'll jump forward and suggest that, if the drug options don't work, then I think it is time for Mom to get some kind of consistent daycare, home care, etc., so that you can have a significant break and rest each and every day and night. The mixture of lack of sleep, getting hit hard and repeatedly, and constant caring for a very demanding and unpredictable patient is no way for you to live. It's dangerous for you, Dad, and we support you in finding other options for continuing to love and support Mom without destroying yourself. I believe Mom would want you to make the best choices for both of you. Figuring out how to do this is priority one, I think.

I cannot imagine how stressful this kind of life must be for you, Dad. I would really hate to have all this stress create such a bad situation that we essentially lose both Mom and Dad simultaneously—I dislike even *writing that sentence out. But that could be what happens as things spiral downwards further with Mom, if there are no good drugs to chill her out, or no regular respite services to give you a big break each day. That is the worst-case scenario that we must avoid at all costs, it seems to me.*

If the drug options are limited or ineffective, then a memory care center such as I believe is being built in Payson right now might need to be the next step. If that one won't be available for a while, then I guess (as frustrating as it might sound) it might be necessary temporarily to relocate Mom (if not both of you) to Tempe or Tucson (if the benefits of staying in Arizona for the insurance money, etc., remain significant). I suspect that getting her to travel even longer distances would be very difficult, if not dangerous at this point, but perhaps she could be relocated to a memory care facility near to one of your two sons and families where you, and several others, could spend significant time with her daily, but not require you to be her primary caregiver constantly.

That's all easier said than done, of course, but for what it's worth, those are my thoughts and advice tonight. Please do let me know if there's anything else I can do to help you out.

In the meantime, very well done again, Dad. You are an amazing husband and a role model Dad!

Love you very much!

[Youngest son]

Now an email from my oldest son:

Dad,

Thank you for asking for our advice. I agree with [youngest son] praising your sacrifices and care for Mom, who by your accounts is less and less herself anymore.

I think we are all beginning to sense that if Mom cannot be effectively medicated soon that she will begin to kill you with abuse, heartbreak and exhaustion. It is very noble and wise to try to take care of Mom yourself as long as possible. However, there are limits to what you can handle and it sounds like you're hitting some of them.

Since Mom is such a pill with you, then I'm worried about what she might do when the kind Payson church ladies pick her up to give you a break. I'd feel terrible if Mom might make one of them cause an auto accident that might hurt people. So unless some medication regime can begin to work, Mom may soon be passing the point where non-professional care can be helpful.

So my suggested plan for you to consider is as follows:

1. Get Mom on a heavy-duty medication program to see if that can chill her out enough that she can stay home with you as you both want without her destroying your life.

2. If what good Alzheimer's doctors prescribe as chill out medication doesn't work, then as [youngest son] also suggests, we need to get Mom admitted into an elder-dementia care facility. This may need to be done to prevent your destruction regardless of whether that is against your and Mom's prior wishes. I don't know if such care is locally available in Payson, but I'm guessing that you can tell [youngest son] and me what you already know about that.

3. When I looked into elder-dementia care facilities in ABQ it was ~$250/day. Please let us know what you've learned about what ALTCS can pay for in AZ to care for Mom.

4. If/when you might need funds beyond what ALTCS can provide, then as long as I remain gainfully employed, [my wife] and I will continue to plan to progressively buy acres of your property to supply you with cash when you need it. We can start soon if you're ready and need it.

Keep your spirits up as best as you can. Go outside, breathe fresh air, look at the stars and keep praying. We all are praying for you here and this trial you are in now shall pass someday.

I'll leave it up to your good judgment if you want to make the trip to ABQ tomorrow for Christmas or not. Either way is OK with us.

Love,

[Oldest son]

My reply to both sons:

[Sons],

Thank you very much for your thoughtful and loving advice. I will continue to look into options for respite care in the home and elsewhere. I spoke to our primary care physician today about the unfortunate consequences of Dee taking the anti-psychotic drug. He said that sometimes happens with all of the sedating medications. One may be tolerated while the next is not. He suggested that I should first start grinding up the Aricept pill that Dee tolerated since the fall of 2011 and putting it into food at suppertime, because calming the patient is one of the characteristic outcomes of using Aricept. He said it might take a week or two to see if it is having the desired effect because she has refused to take any pill for several months. If more of a calming effect would still be desirable he has had success with several other sedative type drugs and would be willing to prescribe one of them. So, that is the course of action that I plan to take.

I decided shortly after I sent you the email this morning that I simply am not up to taking another overnight trip, especially a long one, in Dee's present condition. I am sure she will not be happy with this decision initially, but will benefit from a more relaxed and less stressful schedule. I know I will.

Love,

Dad

Dee was quite jittery the morning and early afternoon of the twenty-third, jumping at my every move or any unusual sound, even on the radio, until a lady friend picked her up just before noon. She remained nervous and afraid of me when the lady and she returned at three thirty. The lady tried to reassure Dee that I am a good guy and love her very much. Dee doubted that and wanted her friend to take her away. Eventually Dee resigned herself to the lady leaving without her. I treated her as gently as I could, but Dee remained jittery as she looked around the house and in closets and drawers as if expecting a bad person to jump out. Trying to divert her attention from this unknown danger, I suggested that we buy some groceries.

Dee helped find items, scooped nuts and granola into plastic sacks, and placed vegetables in the other sacks. She wanted to go straight to bed when we got home but asked why I had only made up her side of the bed. I explained that I had not finished washing and drying sheets to put on my bed. Apparently satisfied, she got undressed, into her pajamas, and into bed. However, she insisted that I remain in the room to protect her from some unseen danger. Fortunately I had a lot of clean sheets and clothes on my side of the bed to fold and put away. Dee soon fell fast asleep. When I finished with that task, I went into the office to read and answer the emails from our two sons. I also attached their emails to the following one I sent to the elder law specialist in Mesa:

To: [Name], Attorney
From: Robert Hershberger
Re: ALTCS
When my wife and I met with you earlier this fall you indicated that it would not be advisable to proceed with an ALTCS application in her current condition. While Dee did not say much that day, she was composed and seemingly self-assured. There has been considerable deterioration in her condition since that time as can be seen in the following series of emails with our two sons. It is best if you read them from bottom to top. I have additional information about changes in her memory, moods and behavior, having kept a written log (now about 60 pages) since we first noticed her memory loss. I also have several photos of bruises and abrasions on my body resulting from her first violent attacks when I tried to lock the office to keep her from removing, misplacing, or even destroying important papers on my desk and in my files.

I have employed a person (on vacation for most of December) to help with housework once a week on Wednesdays and again on Thursday afternoons to provide some respite. I applied for a 5 hour per week respite caregiver *provided by the County Agency on Aging through Catholic Social Services and Lutheran Senior Services. We were granted this respite care after they interviewed my wife and me. However, the first person sent to provide the care was not appreciated by my wife and was, in fact, hit on the back several times by Dee and told to leave when the lady was trying to help Dee with some crafts. I called her supervisor and asked that they discontinue help until January when, hopefully, a more compatible caregiver could be found. I also applied for and received a small respite care grant from the Alzheimer's Association that will provide up to $300 of respite care. We also have a number of women from our church, including the parish nurse, who have known and loved Dee for a number of years that come in occasionally to give me a short break. I could afford on our current income at least another day of respite care each week, but all of these efforts to give me a break are often short circuited by Dee's insistence that I be there with her . . . so my relief has been a maximum of an hour and one half up to this point. Frankly that is not enough. I am getting worn down both physically and emotionally.*

Do you think from reading the correspondence below that it might now be an appropriate time to explore further the ALTCS application and try to protect some of the assets that we have accumulated to enjoy a fuller life in our retirement years?

Please let me know!

Sincerely,

Robert Hershberger

After I completed my exercises and breakfast in the morning, I called a friend in Phoenix to obtain the name and number of her contact at Payson Hospice and told her about all that had happened after we left the marvelous *White Christmas* stage play.

I called hospice and left my number, doubting that I would hear back from them until after Christmas. Dee was still in bed at eleven thirty this Christmas Eve morning. I had hoped that she would get up happy so we could enjoy Christmas Eve and Christmas together in our home. But she got up in a bad mood with her frequent mantra that she has no clothes. Her mood completely changed when I brought out her entire outfit, right down to appropriate jewelry. I told her about going to the Christmas Eve service and she liked the idea. I also asked if she would like me to wash her hair. She did, so I washed her hair before helping her put on the outfit. She seemed happy but jumped every time I moved or she heard something. She ate all of her breakfast with a little coaxing and drank a little bit of juice and some water. It pleased me to see her eating again because she had lost an additional 15 pounds between September and December. She now weighs only 110 pounds after maintaining a weight of 135 pounds for many years.

The social worker at hospice called back before long and arranged for an admissions person to evaluate Dee. The promptness of her response pleased me. The admissions person came at one thirty and after a thorough evaluation of Dee concluded that hospice services were warranted, so I signed the necessary paperwork. Hospice services include Dee receiving several days in their facility to allow me some needed respite, covered by Medicare. So another piece of the care puzzle is finally in place. Their social service person and nurse will visit Thursday to determine if Dee qualifies for ALTCS given her current capabilities and behavior.

On Christmas morning Dee ate her breakfast, then suddenly jumped up and ran to the bathroom but did not make it. So like so many times before, I had her pajamas, bottom, some of the floor, and the toilet to clean. She allowed me to clean her bottom, wash her face and body, and brush her teeth without any fuss and accepted my choice of clothes, including a new blouse. But she became angry that she could not be with our sons for Christmas when we opened presents. She talked about going home to her mother and many other impossible scenarios and said, "I'll walk home." She jumped up and left the house in a rush, but feeling cold outside she soon came back. However, she remained in a very dark mood and did not like any gift she opened.

Our oldest son called as I took hamburgers off the grill for lunch so we talked to him and his family while eating. The call calmed Dee quite a bit, so I suggested that we go out and enjoy the beautiful weather. We did for a little while. When we returned, I made Dee a root beer float and she drank most of it, but then she became fidgety and even aggressive for no apparent reason. I asked if she would like soup for dinner. She nodded that she would and supervised its preparation. But when I put it on the table, she wanted to go to bed. It is hard to stay pleasant under these circumstances so I became grumpy about leaving the warm food on the table.

As I tucked her into bed, Dee declared, "I will die tonight."

"I doubt it," I replied.

"You must hate me!" she cried.

"Not true. I love you!" I assured her.

I gave her a kiss on the cheek, turned off the lights, and left the room. I think she went to sleep immediately. This is a Christmas that I will remember, but not fondly.

THURSDAY, DECEMBER 26, 2013 ॐ

The hospice social worker and the registered nurse came at ten this morning and asked good questions. Dee enjoyed having them in our home and sang Christmas songs with the caseworker while the nurse and I talked. I liked what she told me about their services. The social worker said that the Mesa attorney would prepare legal documents for Dee's acceptance into the state's long-term care system and that Dee's symptoms definitely will allow her to qualify medically. She wants to stay in the loop and indicated that we were wise not to buy long-term care insurance because insurance companies make the conditions for care so terminal and waiting periods so long that almost no one receives a dime from these companies. This did not surprise me because I knew from experience that insurance companies in the construction field always find ways to avoid payouts.

The nurse took Dee's vital signs and found her to be very healthy physically. We discussed alternative treatments for Dee's extreme anxiety and violent outbursts. The nurse said that lorazepam might work as a mild sedative and that Depakote might work for aggressive behavior. I told them about the advice our family doctor gave about restarting Aricept ground up in food because of its mild palliative effect. They agreed and gave me their direct telephone numbers so I could call at any time. The nurse took a copy of my diary as background information. She indicated that she would visit Dee weekly on Mondays between ten and noon. I said that I would contact the attorney to prepare the legal documents needed to obtain health care for Dee.

We received calls during lunch from a certified nursing assistant (CNA) about seeing us at four that afternoon about the services she could provide and from the hospice chaplain about seeing us on Friday morning at ten. I am really impressed with how quickly hospice responds.

Dee got really angry with me in the afternoon and began to lash out with her fists and feet. I kept my distance, telling her, "Honey, I don't like getting hit!" About that time the CNA arrived, but Dee insisted that she leave immediately. Thankfully Dee did not hit or kick her. I made arrangements for the lady to come on Wednesday mornings at ten, the time of day when Dee is usually in a better mood. Due to Dee's rush to get the CNA to leave, I failed to get her business card and can't remember her name. My hope is that she can help Dee with her hair, nails, and the like.

Dee remained in a foul mood through dinner and refused to eat the split pea soup in which I put the ground-up Aricept. It was not the taste of the Aricept that she did not like because Dee refused even to take a sip. Eventually I got her to drink a quarter of a glass of milk and eat a slice of multigrain toast with butter and some coffee ice cream, in which I placed another ground-up Aricept pill. I am really stressed out.

FRIDAY, DECEMBER 27, 2013 ஃ
This was another day of many mood changes. Dee woke up with me at about eight and agreed to take a shower and wash her hair. We did this without a negative incident and she readily put on the clothes that I laid

out for her. We ate breakfast and looked forward to meeting the hospice chaplain. He is a big, jolly person with a pleasant smile. Dee related well to him as he asked us questions. He brought his guitar and had a sing-along with Dee of familiar tunes. We agreed to have him come every Wednesday afternoon at two to pray and sing with Dee, and me when I am available. I think this will provide a good break in the day. (Actually, he never returned. I'm not sure why.)

I made Canadian bacon and avocado sandwiches, once a favorite of Dee's, for lunch. She took a few bites and refused to eat any more, saying, "They taste awful." She also said she would not eat the leftover split pea soup. So I threw it out—a hard thing for a Depression baby to do. Dee did agree to eat some ice cream and drink some water. I should have put the Aricept in the ice cream because she refused to eat the blueberry pancakes that I made for dinner. (Now I know how homemakers feel when family members will not eat what they prepare. I really admire their patience.)

Throughout the early evening Dee threatened and hit me when she could. Then she apologized and said she would be good. She went into the bedroom, shut the door, and told me to stay out. I did until she came out and begged me to help her get ready for bed. I helped her into bed without cleaning up. I cannot express how nerve-racking this behavior is to me. I am thankful that it happens early so I can have a quiet evening to myself.

MONDAY, DECEMBER 30, 2013 ᅇ

Today Dee was the best I have seen her in several months. She seemed happy and calm from the time she got up. The hospice nurse came at about ten thirty and had a good time with Dee while taking her vitals and talking with her. We showed her Dee's artwork and paintings. The nurse seemed truly impressed. She asked if I would consider using any anxiety medication. I said if every day was like today, I would say no. But given the previous week, I agreed that I should. So the nurse said she would contact Dee's doctor to see if Depakote in flake form would be an appropriate medication.

The parish nurse from our church came in the afternoon to take Dee to a movie and for ice cream. Dee sat through *The Secret Life of Walter Mitty* and for an ice cream dish afterward with no aggravation. They came home full of smiles. Dee and I then ran errands, bought groceries, and enjoyed a deli dinner. Once home Dee helped put away the groceries then went right to bed. It was a wonderful day.

TUESDAY, DECEMBER 31, 2013 ᆇ

What a roller coaster! Dee awoke very cranky, jumpy, and fearful of every sound, apparently imagining the worst. She resisted being washed, brushing her teeth, and getting dressed. She grudgingly accompanied me on a short walk but saw everything along the way as either something wonderful . . . or something terrible and threatening.

When we got home Dee flew into a rage and threw a whole bunch of my folders on the floor, swept a glass off my desk, and pummeled me when I asked her to stop. I retreated into the kitchen and to the other side of the counters to keep my distance while she tried to catch me. Finally she apologized and said she would be nice. But then she began looking around the house for something or someone threatening her. I am sure she saw things that were not there because she screamed, jumped, cried, and whimpered through it all.

Dee wanted to go to bed at six but she would not get in bed unless I did. So I invited her back to the office to read my emails. She came in but became frantic and said she would sleep in the office and sat down on the floor. This lasted a few minutes, until she got cold and insisted that we both go to bed.

"I won't force you to go to bed and you can't force me to go to bed," I told her.

She replied clearly, "I have a bad headache."

"When I have a bad headache, I go to bed," I responded.

Finally, at about six thirty, she headed for the bedroom, but she soon came back to ask for help. I helped her take off her clothes and put on her pajamas, tucked her into bed, and gave her a big hug, kiss, and assurances that I love her.

When I went to bed at about ten thirty it was as if New Year's Eve never occurred.

Reflections on the Third Year ə♥

When 2013 began, I still had a loving wife and hope that Alzheimer's could be cured or would progress slowly and not affect Dee the way it apparently did many others. I was not prepared emotionally for what happened later in the year.

I knew that Dee's ability to cope would decline and that she would become confused, but the signs of some kind of psychosis in which she saw and feared things not present surprised me. She became jumpy and scared about almost anything. But, most surprising and hurtful, literally and figuratively, was her violent behavior toward me. Being larger and stronger, I could defend myself and even hold her down until her violent behavior subsided. But I could not control my emotions. I could not accept that the person who loved me so much could treat me so badly. It hurt too much. Now, reflecting on what made her behave this way, I wonder if I could have stopped this behavior by smiling, laughing, and even joking when she tried to hurt me. At the time, I simply did not have the emotional strength to do it.

I now understand the desperation that caused me to search for a magical cure to this horrendous disease and also, unfortunately, that some medical professionals prey on people like me with false claims of cure.

I also understand that an outside project that a caregiver must complete can be misunderstood by a person with Alzheimer's and become a source of great pain. Ideally, caregivers would be in a position to provide undivided attention to their loved ones to keep them from becoming distraught. This, of course, is unrealistic. Caregivers must have some distractions and time for personal activities to avoid going crazy. It was important to have Dee's friends relieve me from time to time.

Alzheimer's disease, while a mental disorder, doesn't just stop there. The mind controls all bodily functions, so the ability to do physical activities declines and, even more problematic, control of bodily functions wanes. Incontinence becomes a major issue, and cleanup can be a very messy, stinky activity. The person with Alzheimer's may also become very stubborn about wearing something to absorb urine. But more problematic, especially with women, fecal incontinence increases the likelihood of urinary tract or vaginal infection. And persons with Alzheimer's may have no ability to describe to a caregiver the origin of their pain—pain that often causes aggressive behavior.

Worst of all is the day when your loved one no longer knows who you are. It is devastating, especially when you become the "very bad man" (or woman). You have no idea how much that hurts until it happens to you. Fortunately, in my case, recognition came and went, so at least Dee recognized me and wanted me near most of the time.

Advice to Caregivers ҉

1. Pray that your loved one continues to have a pleasant personality for the duration of the disease. But if this prayer goes unanswered and your loved one becomes very difficult, try to get him or her into a safe environment where you and/or someone else can provide care in a loving and safe way. I strongly recommend someone else if you cannot physically or emotionally handle your loved one. I cannot imagine how a small person could care for a combative large person. It would be an extremely dangerous proposition.

2. Be prepared to deal with a loved one with some kind of psychosis, imagining all kinds of horrendous things and as a result pleading with you to kill them or help them kill themselves. I told Dee that I could not do this because of the law, but it was also because I could not imagine doing either thing to or with her. Use some kind of diversion to get the person to focus on something else. But with your response always try to show your love. Your loved one really is experiencing these awful things.

3. Don't waste your time reading stories or advertisements about miracle cures for Alzheimer's disease. They are scams. Stick with advice from credible organizations like the Alzheimer's Association and the medical professionals in your community.

4. If you are in a position to do so, unload your professional, service, or social obligations onto someone else. Especially try to avoid projects that consume your time. You will find that your loved one needs all of your time and attention to assure them both of your love and that you will not leave them. It is hard to imagine beforehand how needy the person with Alzheimer's will become.

5. These final years with my wife would have been so much better if I had not been trying to finish a project outside our home. Dee needed the constant attention and loving care that I could not provide while completing the cabin in New Mexico. I advise you to have someone else look after such projects if you want your loved one to remain happy with you. If possible, put all expensive projects on hold. A large project requiring the expenditure of financial resources can take away your ability to pay for services needed to care for your loved one.

6. If you haven't already done so, start finding social service agencies that can provide caregivers to support you. Home care can quickly eat up your financial resources as the need becomes greater. Apply for Medicaid-type support if you do not have enough money to provide this care over a period of years. You will need the help of friends,

relatives, or hired caregivers even to find the necessary time to complete an application for such support.

7. Reach out to friends and family for assistance. A special friend of Dee's from our church seemed like a gift sent from God when she began arranging for a variety of Dee's women friends from our church to come two at a time to take her out to a movie and for treats some afternoons. This gave me a much needed two- to three-hour break, and their smiling faces and happy chatter usually left Dee in a much better mood when she returned home.

8. Try to prepare for the day when your loved one no longer knows who you are, and especially when the person thinks you are an intruder, in my case a "very bad man." It is extremely difficult to accept this from someone you love and who loved you for many years.

9. If your loved one feels safe in some activity, make a special effort to keep him or her involved with it. My wife loved going to church. It was always the high point of the week and the only time when she did not become difficult or combative with me or anyone else. I often wished that every day could be Sunday.

4

Fourth Year
of the Journey

৵

The new year did not bring improvement in Dee's ability, mood, or behavior. She is often in a state of near panic, especially in the late afternoons and early evenings before she finally falls asleep. She goes through periods of anxiety, depression, desire to die, and fear that someone or something will hurt her or us. She jumps anytime she hears an unfamiliar noise on the radio or TV and even fears that I might kill her. She is experiencing something truly terrifying.

Dee awakened at eight last night and came into the office insisting that I go to bed with her. Noticing the fear in her eyes, I did. She clung tightly to me until she fell asleep. I slept until five in the morning and planned to get up, when Dee suddenly sat up and called out, "Mom."

"I'm next to you," I replied.

She took my hand and fell asleep. I remained wide-awake until a quarter to six, when I got up to finish this entry.

The next day we picked up a prescription of Depakote at the drugstore. It comes in little capsules that can be taken apart and the contents sprinkled on food.

My anxiety level went way up for the next three days because Dee took only two pills on the food I sprinkled with Depakote. She says it tastes bad. I am sure it does. So I called the hospice nurse, who told me to discontinue the drug for now because I'm so anxious and frustrated.

THURSDAY, JANUARY 9, 2014 ᳱ

Dee continues to have episodes of anxiety and fear, with the worst episode today on the way home from a pleasant visit with my cousin and her husband in Apache Junction. Dee had been fidgety and fearful all day, but while driving back to Payson after dark she jerked uncontrollably, kicked the dashboard, and hit the door and me. I think she was trying to chase away demons. She jerked my right hand away from the steering wheel once, but I maintained control of the car with my left hand. I feared that she might jerk both hands from the steering wheel and cause us to crash, so I clung tightly to the wheel and we made it home.

FRIDAY, JANUARY 10, 2014 ᳱ

"I don't like her," Dee said when a young caregiver came to help with crafts. We let her in but she made us uncomfortable as she watched us finish lunch. Dee lightened up a bit on a long walk with her and me after lunch and treated her civilly while doing crafts.

Dee seemed happy, even jolly, and ate everything at supper. She agreed to watch TV and cuddled up beside me to watch the news. About a half hour into the program she began to make advances, kissing me on the neck, cheeks, and lips. I was so hungry for her love that I could hardly stand it. Before long, she insisted that we go to bed and make love. I had hoped that we would do this again sometime, so I readily agreed. We walked hand in hand to the bedroom and made love. She seemed like the normal lover of our previous years of marriage. I felt like I had died and gone to Heaven because I waited so long to share my love with her again. What a change! Unbelievable! We fell sound asleep under the covers in the nude.

I awoke around midnight to go to the bathroom and put on my pajamas before awakening Dee to use the toilet and put on hers. She remembered nothing about making love but seemed happy when I tucked her back into bed with a tender kiss. I then spent some time wondering about what had happened in her brain to make this possible. I guess I will never know.

SATURDAY, JANUARY 11, 2014 ৯৬
Dee was equally happy this morning when we went grocery shopping. She ate well at lunch and we had a really good time in the afternoon with me practicing golf and her watching. She exhibited no signs of anxiety, fear, or anger. Indeed, Dee tried to communicate her thoughts about pleasant things throughout the day. I listened intently and indicated that I understood. Her happy smile and bright eyes returned. I love it and wonder if Dee has entered a new phase of the disease. Is a miracle happening? Is the disease in retreat? I hope so!

TUESDAY, JANUARY 14, 2014 ৯৬
I wrote nothing about what happened on Sunday and Monday. Both days must have been mostly good. In other words, there must have been no bad news, headlines, or disasters. Imagine that. Four good days in a row!

The good news ceased today. Dee became impatient and angry with me as I prepared lunch. She wanted her food immediately. After lunch a certified nursing assistant (CNA) arrived to help Dee bathe, wash her hair, and prepare food for tomorrow's lunch. I planned to stay home the first hour while Dee and the lady became acquainted, then to practice golf during the warmest part of the day and get a haircut.

Dee did not want the lady to stay and was uncooperative, belligerent, and threatening immediately after I left. So when I got home just before five, the lady indicated that she had accomplished little because of Dee's unwillingness to cooperate and frequent attempts to leave the house. She also indicated that it would not be possible for her or anyone to care for Dee if her moods and behavior were not better controlled. She said that hospice should prescribe medication to calm Dee's anxiety and mellow her temper and behavior. She also suggested that I place Dee in the hospice care facility for a week or so to get her stabilized. "That will give you time to do something unrelated to caregiving to help relieve your stress." I left a message for the hospice nurse to call and tell me what to do. I hope she does because I am at my wits' end.

FRIDAY, JANUARY 24, 2014 ❧

Over a week has passed and I managed to have Dee take her pills daily. She hallucinates less but still sees and talks to people who are not there. On walks she tries to go into houses in the neighborhood to see people we do not know. But she has not been terrified like when we drove home from Apache Junction after a dinner with my cousin and her husband. Several days this week Dee broke into tears and repeated the mantra, "You don't like me," even after I replied, "I like you and love you very much." But she undoubtedly reads my body language. The constant questions and incessant crying annoy me. I am sure it shows.

SUNDAY, JANUARY 26, 2014 ❧

We got up at eight this morning after Dee grabbed my little finger so hard I thought it would break. Amazingly we got to church a bit early. Dee greeted her friends with warm hugs and "I love you" while I enjoyed talking with these same friends. Church went well. Afterward several people decided to go to lunch with us. Dee became increasingly agitated, especially with me, when the food did not come immediately. When it came, I asked a lady to comfort Dee so I could eat. At first Dee refused to eat anything, but the lady coaxed her into eating toast that I had sprinkled with Depakote. Dee then insisted on leaving, so I apologized to the others and we came home.

FRIDAY, JANUARY 31, 2014 ॐ

I noticed something new today. Dee was unsteady and slow while ascending the stairs. In the past, she often ran up the steps two at a time with no hand on the rail. Something is going on that makes her less steady. She is less interested in exercise and in taking walks at any speed. I do not allow her to carry anything on the stairs now because of her observable unsteadiness. She struggles just to get her body up or down the stairs.

My life is now mostly miserable because I see little chance of having caregivers watch over Dee when I am out. I feel trapped and angry about what is happening to Dee and to me. I hope there will be some relief in the near future.

WEDNESDAY, FEBRUARY 5, 2014 ॐ

Dee's behavior continues as usual. By about three in the afternoon, something sets her off and makes her violent. Today she got very upset about something and began hitting and chasing me around. She picked up a book and hit me with it on the arm that I used to shield my face and body. She started to kick at me as I moved away, then picked up a stool and swung it at me. I grabbed the stool to stop her, but she lunged at me and we tumbled onto a swivel rocking chair and tipped a floor lamp over onto the dining table. The impact broke one of the light bulbs and its support. Dee continued hitting me, so I retreated to my dressing room. She followed, commanding me to get out of the house. When I wouldn't leave, she said she would and stormed out of the house. I called the social worker to tell her what had happened as I went after Dee. I found her about two blocks away, very cold and ready to return home. We walked hand in hand back to the house, but once inside she became violent again. I dashed toward the bedroom with her close behind. When she would not relent, I wrestled her onto the bed and held her down in a way that she could not hit, bite, or kick me. Finally she relaxed, so I let her up. We returned to the dining room, where I cleaned up the broken glass. Dee seemed remorseful but could not remember what happened.

The hospice nurse called and we discussed the possibility of placing Dee at the hospice facilities for a week or in a wing for violent persons at a local nursing home. She said no to the hospice facilities because they are not equipped to handle violent behavior but that she would try to make arrangements at a local care facility. She also suggested using a quick-acting gel to calm Dee. While the nurse and I talked, Dee left the house and walked about two blocks away. She apparently decided to return home, so I met her coming back and asked her to return home with me. She seemed happy and surprised to see me and came home peaceably.

SATURDAY, FEBRUARY 8, 2014 ৯৵

Our morning began peacefully but with Dee insisting that she would soon have a baby. A baby! I tried to talk with her about this rationally regarding her age and menopause but to no avail. She was convinced. She would soon have a baby. But it did not arrive. When we went golfing in the very nice afternoon weather, Dee rode along happily in the golf cart and never suggested that we had to go or do anything else. I relaxed and played well, and we enjoyed milkshakes on the way home. By four thirty she was ready for a bit of soup and toast and I got the medication into her. I heard no more about the baby and she went to bed without any fuss. Weird!

TUESDAY, FEBRUARY 11, 2014 ৯৵

Dee enjoyed having the CNA wash and style her hair on Monday while the nurse and I talked about a week of respite care at the end of the month. I gave Dee her first dose of a calming medication today but observed no calming. She was hyperactive with the parish nurse in the afternoon, so much so that the nurse called afterward and said that I must get all scissors and knives under lock and key. She worries about Dee throwing something hard at me or at the glass doors and mirrors. I share these concerns but have no idea how to correct the situation. There are glass doors on nearly every cabinet and no locks on kitchen drawers.

SUNDAY, FEBRUARY 23, 2014 ৵

Dee got up early with me so we could take showers and get ready for church. However, she first took a dump in a wastebasket by the bedroom door. It must have looked like a toilet to her, or at least close enough. So I cleaned up the mess before we took our showers. After she finished showering I helped her get dressed, but it upset her when I tried to finish my shower and get dressed. We got to church in time for Sunday school and she sat and listened quietly. She also did well in church.

MONDAY, FEBRUARY 24, 2014 ৵

I took Dee to the nursing home at ten thirty this morning. She had no problem until she saw her room, and then she went ballistic. She grabbed her already open suitcase and stormed toward the door with clothes falling out along the way. I rescued the suitcase and clothes while the nurse followed Dee to the locked doors of the unit. Dee came back into the room just steaming, grabbed some of her clothes, and rushed out again with the nursing staff close behind. She did not calm down after I left, even after they applied a soothing gel and gave her a calming drug. I went home feeling bad about putting her in the facility but knowing I need time to complete the Arizona Long Term Care Service (ALTCS) application, something I cannot do with Dee constantly taking and misplacing items and generally disrupting me. On the way home I heard "Somewhere over the Rainbow" playing on the radio and broke out in tears that would not stop. There is no foreseeable rainbow in our lives. I am about as sad as I have ever been.

TUESDAY, FEBRUARY 25, 2014 ৵

I stopped by the care center today and talked with the head nurse, who said that Dee had not responded well to the drugs and requires constant one-on-one attention, something they are not prepared to offer. He said they would keep her until Saturday as agreed to with hospice but she could not come back for a second respite to allow me to prepare income tax returns.

I have most of the ALTCS material ready for a meeting with the attorney on Thursday but still need some material from New Mexico. It will take all day tomorrow to get everything else organized and request the missing items. I will then drive to Mesa to meet with the attorney and attend an Alzheimer's conference to learn "How to Deal with Difficult Behaviors." My, how I need this advice!

I feel like Dee and I are in hell. It is no fun for either of us. I am sad that she has to stay in a place she hates for five days. I wonder how she will respond when I pick her up on Saturday morning and do not look forward to catching the brunt of her anger. I wonder how I will prepare taxes this year with her in the house. I am desperate but with no good way out of this mess.

THURSDAY, FEBRUARY 27, 2014 ❧

I worked diligently Monday through Wednesday collecting and copying the information required by the elder care attorney and finished late Wednesday night, except for one piece of information from Social Security that I have to obtain from their Mesa office. However, I received a call from the hospice social worker when driving to Mesa on Thursday saying, "You must pick up Dee today, not Saturday. The nursing home cannot handle Dee without a full-time CNA at her side, which is more than they bargained for." So I canceled lunch and dinner with friends, forgot about golf, canceled my hotel reservation, informed the leader of our Alzheimer's support group that I would not attend the conference, and went to the Social Security office. It took an hour and three quarters for the Social Security personnel to get to my case, but once in the booth it took only a few minutes to become Dee's surrogate and obtain the required form. That left five minutes to get to the attorney's office without having lunch. After two hours with the attorneys and their legal assistants, I purchased a beef sandwich and cookie at a nearby fast-food place and headed for Payson. I called and talked with both of our boys on the way home and agreed to fill them in later in the evening.

Dee was sleeping when I got to the nursing home, so I packed her suitcase, filled out paperwork, got her drugs, and tried to wake her up. The drugs they used had put her into a stupor. I felt so sad and guilty seeing her in this condition. I do not like her being treated this way. Her slacks were wet with urine and she smelled from a dump in her adult diapers. She looked awful. I felt awful.

I feel so ashamed for having left Dee to this fate. I had already decided to do everything I can for her at home, devoting one-on-one all day, every day to try to keep her happy and noncombative. I'll do my best until I know this approach isn't working. I'll let Dee sleep as long as she can tonight and into the morning. Then I will try to clean her bottom, give her a shower, wash her hair, and get rid of any remnant of her stay at the nursing home. I am just plain emotionally exhausted and can see no respite in the future. They say God gives you no more than you can handle. How would they know? I've reached my limit. Dee has exceeded hers.

FRIDAY, FEBRUARY 28–WEDNESDAY, MARCH 5, 2014 ❧
I received the following email from my sister on the twenty-eighth:

Bob,

I read several articles this morning on the Internet about the various stages of Alzheimer's and how to deal with patients who have anger issues. One of the things they stressed was the need for caregivers to get time for themselves, which was why you had Dee go to that local facility. I know you don't want Dee over medicated, sleeping all the time, or acting like a zombie, but at the same time you have to be in shape, mentally and physically, to take care of her. The problem is how to achieve that goal. It seems to me that some sort of compromise is in order. Perhaps more medication than you want her to

have for a short 4- or 5-day period every month or so, while you take care of
personal needs and business issues. Please consider it.

Your good emotional and physical health is at stake, Bob. Without that,
Dee will not have the care you want for her.

My thoughts and prayers are with you and Dee every day.

Much love,

[Sister]

Then followed several emails with family over the next few days, starting
with two replies to my sister:

[Sister],

I appreciate your concern and advice. It is the same I am getting from about
everyone. But there are some other considerations. I was supposed to take
a 5-day respite period this week. I worked feverishly on a 30-item list of
ALTCS information day and night, Monday through Wednesday. This was
not respite. But I did get it done! Thursday morning early I headed to Mesa
to get required information from the Social Security office. But I was called
on Thursday morning (while waiting 1¾ hours to be served at the SS offices)
by the Hospice social worker telling me that I had to return to Payson and
pick up Dee from the care center. Dee was apparently so hyper that they
had to assign a CNA to her constantly to protect her and other people in
the lockdown ward. Medicare does not pay for this level of care, at least
at this care center. I told the social worker that I would come immediately
after meeting with the lawyers about the Arizona Long Term Care System
(ALTCS), arriving in Payson between 5 and 6 p.m. I had to cancel a lunch
with five very good friends from University Presbyterian days, a golf game
in the late afternoon, dinner with my ex-partner (and his wife) and hotel
reservations. I also had to cancel my attendance at an Alzheimer's conference
with several noted persons having sessions relating to difficult behaviors and
the like. I will be getting a CD on all of the presentations so all is not lost. So,
in 3½ days I got zero respite.

Dee was fast asleep on her bed at the care center with a CNA sitting beside her when I got there. She smelled of urine and poop and her pants were wet. So, I packed her suitcase, took care of check out, and endeavored to wake her up. The nurse on duty came in to assist me and we eventually had her up onto a wheelchair. I was assisted by the CNA and another aide getting her into the Prius. At home I carefully sleep walked her up the stairs into the bedroom and placed her on the La-Z-Boy recliner, covered her up, and let her sleep until 4 in the morning when she awoke and wanted to go to the bathroom. I took her in and she had what looked like at least two days of excrement and urine in her adult diapers. It took me more than half an hour to clean her up and get the soiled clothes off. I then took her into the shower to wash her from top to bottom, as it was apparent that no one washed her in the three days at the care center. She proceeded to dump standing up with my constant support as she was ¾ asleep. I picked up the droppings and dropped them into the toilet. I dried her and got on clean panties and pajamas and put her in her regular bed, where she was soon fast asleep. I then took my shower and went back to bed at 5:30 a.m. I woke up at 6:30 a.m. and did my yoga exercises until Dee awoke at 7:30 wanting to go to the bathroom. She had more dump in her panties and on her bottom that I proceeded to clean up. She was groggy all day and unable to control her bowel movements so I did the same thing three more times, washing lots of clothes and towels in between.

Well, that's a long and not so pretty story, but the result of Dee being given a sedating medication that left her in a stupor from about 11 a.m. on Thursday until mid-morning today. She came out of the complete stupor but was groggy all day and has not regained control of her bowel function. She also could no longer walk standing straight up as she always had until she went into the care center. She was bent over at the waist and shuffled her feet all throughout the day today. She was not angry or mean, just foggy and impatient at times.

I decided not to give her any more medication, at least over the weekend, hoping to allow the "poison" medicines to get out of her system; hoping beyond hope that she will at least return to her condition before the 3+ days at the care center to where she can walk upright, not shuffle and know when bowel movements are coming. We'll see if this "detox" works.

So, suppose in another month I take her to another care center. I certainly will not return to this one. How much capacity will she lose there? How much harder will it be for me to care for her at home? Today was hard. I kept my cool and treated her with love and affection throughout, but found her hiding from me several times. When asked why she was hiding she expressed in her limited way that she was afraid I might hurt her. She has bruises on her right biceps where someone at the care center had obviously grabbed her very tightly trying to get her to behave before she was sedated. I am sure she knew in some visceral way that I had left her at the center and gone away. So, she had reason to associate me with hurtful behavior.

I am hoping that by taking her off all or at least most medications and by treating her with love and respect, never anger or harsh words, that she will calm down on her own and maintain better control of bodily functions. And maybe I can get some respite care workers to come and be with her while I do work needing to be done or get out to practice golf, play tennis, bicycle or even take a long vigorous walk. Here again we will see.

Meanwhile it will take six to eight months to get approval from ALTCS to get up to 30 hours of in home care for Dee or (if it must be) full time care in a licensed Alzheimer's care facility. Meanwhile, I cannot sell our home or afford to have Dee stay in such a facility with a $75,000 to $100,000 per year price tag. So, at least until then, Dee and I will be staying here in Payson in our home. I doubt that I will want to take another chance on a brief stay at a care center . . . only one other one in town. So . . . ?

If Dee is accepted into ALTCS then I would be able to sell the house and we could move into an apartment or an independent or assisted living facility; somewhere where I would no longer have to be involved with housekeeping, meal preparation, gardening and the like. It would also be more likely in this setting that I could get a woman caregiver to come in for a week or so while I got away to do something on my own . . . skiing, fishing, golfing, etc. etc.

*I have also sent this email to [my brother and children] knowing that all
of you are concerned about both Dee's and my welfare.*

*I love all of you very much and really do appreciate your concerns and I
am open to suggestions.*

Love,

Bob

[Sister],

*Sorry I was so peevish last night. I suppose it was because I was both tired
and peeved. Please forgive.*

*Today was much better. Dee woke up with me refreshed and willing to
try some yoga poses before getting distracted. She started out bent over with
the shuffle, but by the end of the day walked with me to the library and back
standing erect and gradually picking up speed on the way home. Yes! She
was back to her usual one bowel movement in the morning and had only
one accident. MOST important she was back to her more normal loving
personality. I think that no pills are going to work best! Hope this continues.*

Love,

Bob

On March 2 I tried to bring everyone up to date:

[Everyone],

*Today was totally unlike yesterday. Dee got up very hyper and has remained
so all day. She did pretty well at church greeting everyone several times and
singing even with the choir during the service. At communion she grabbed
the half loaf of bread from the server and took off a big chunk, then bolted
toward the back of the church with me close behind. Fortunately, the server
grabbed the half loaf back before Dee took off. Later in the service Dee
decided we had to go home right now, which we did. She was difficult at
lunch, getting up and down several times and dropping food on the floor*

before leaving for good to sit down on the floor inside her closet. I think she sensed a need for a time out. Somewhere along the way she had a bowel movement, which took lots of time to clean up . . . a mess. Since then she has been erratic and combative.

While this was going on I called [sister] so she experienced some of the background excitement. She had been thinking about the situation and talked to the director of a very good elder care facility near her home. He suggested that Dee needed to be placed for at least 5 days in the psychiatric section of a high quality Alzheimer's unit in which they could work to get the medications right. He suggested such a facility was at [major hospital] in Phoenix.

I will be talking to the Hospice nurse on Monday morning about this and other possible ways to get a handle on how to care for Dee.

Thanks again for all of your good advice and prayers. We need both.

Love,

Bob

My brother's response and my reply on the third:

Bob,

We just want you to know that we have been monitoring the family emails, and have had several conversations with [sister]. We love both you and Dee and you are in our prayers. It is a difficult time for both of you! For Dee because she is, perhaps, not the Dee that we all knew, and who has lost her understanding. For you, because you have that understanding and are doing all (more than all perhaps) that is humanly possible. Please take care and get the help out there that is possible. In the long term, I am afraid that [father-in-law's] long-term care resulted in the death of [mother-in-law]. We do not want something like that to happen here.

If it is a matter of dollars. We can help. We love you.

[Brother]

[Brother],

Thank you very much for your concern and generous financial offer. I hope it will be possible to care for Dee here at home until the ALTCS application runs its course . . . 5 to 8 months if past applications are an indicator. If it works we should be able to get plenty of care here at home (if Dee ceases to be so difficult behaviorally). If not, we would be able to place her in a facility with staff prepared to deal with such behavior . . . probably by sedating her to a level that I find appalling. If we are unsuccessful because we have too many assets, we would probably have to sell and spend them down to the point where Dee can qualify. Nursing care in a facility around here runs $6,500 per month and up for specialized care. This would take nearly all of our current retirement income so simply is not feasible. If we were able to sell all of our real estate assets at a reasonable rate we could probably pay for such care for 5 or 6 years before running out of assets and definitely becoming eligible for ALTCS. We'll just have to see what transpires with the application and hope that Dee's disposition will make it possible to live together until then.

I am doing pretty well so far but could use more time on my own when the stress gets high. I think the only feasible way to do this would be to have someone or someones Dee knows and loves come to our home and be with her when I am gone. I have not found anyone in a position to do this up until now.

Thank you very much for your love and concern.

Love,

Bob

Another email to my brother on the fourth:

[Brother],

Monday was a gloriously happy day with Dee very mellow, bright eyed, and friendly throughout the day. The Hospice nurse came to assess Dee and agreed with my suggestion that Sunday's rather bizarre behavior was probably at least partly the result of Dee's withdrawing from the anti-psychotic medicine she had been taking. The CNA was able to wash and style Dee's hair and Dee was elated with how she looked afterwards. Then two good women friends came with lunch sandwiches and spent the early afternoon with Dee while I went to the bank to prepare changes in accounts to help make it possible for Dee to qualify for ALTCS, Arizona's long term care program. The women reported that they had a wonderful time with Dee looking over all of the diaries that [youngest son] and [youngest grandson] prepared and some of the Christmas memory books that Dee had prepared. The rest of day was very pleasant.

Today started out the same way and lasted through lunch when Dee became very excited about a visit from another good woman friend that arrived late. Dee just couldn't wait and became very stressed and took it out on me. But once the lady arrived, our parish nurse, Dee was happy again and the two of them went out to walk around the lake at Green Valley Park to look at the birds and sang hymns together in the lady's car. I worked on the ALTCS materials while they were gone. When they came home, Dee was very happy to see me and suggested that we have a party. So we opened a sparkling apple grape drink and the three of us enjoyed conversation at the table for over an hour. I made the mistake of waiting too long for dinner so Dee became agitated. I have to be more careful about time management!

Overall, I am pleased with the direction we are going and so is Dee. I hope it continues in this direction.

Love,

Bob

An email from my sister and my reply on the fifth:

Bob,

I'm so glad to hear that Dee is doing better and able to enjoy having people come to visit. That gives you a much needed break in the daily routine and makes life ever so much more enjoyable,

What is the status on her meds? Did you discuss with the nurse the possibility of a hospital stay at a "geropsych" unit to determine the appropriate levels and types of medication for her?

I hope today is another good day.

Much love to you both.

[Sister]

[Sister],

Since I picked her up on Thursday evening, Dee has been on no medications. Her mood has varied from rather benign and loving to mean and impatient except for the withdrawal day on Sunday. Today she was mostly mean and impatient.

The nurse and I decided to try for a week to see how Dee does on no medication. Then we will discuss options for medicine if Dee's behavior warrants it. We will not go back on Aricept because it has outlived its usefulness in delaying short-term memory loss. It is gone. And Aricept may have been contributing to Dee's behavioral issues. We will not go back onto Depakote because, if anything, it increased her psychotic behavior as the dosage increased. We may try very small doses of the Ativan that really knocked her out on Thursday and Friday. If this does not work we discussed a couple of options for a "geropsych" hospital stay in Phoenix. The nurse said [major hospital's] behavioral unit was not strictly geriatric and felt a different facility aimed only at elderly would be better for Dee. So, I will know more in a week or so.

Again, I appreciate your concern and advice!

Love,

Bob

THURSDAY, MARCH 6, 2014 ❧

Great day! I gave Dee my undivided attention all day and it paid off. We showered and washed hair before breakfast. She was happy all morning and enjoyed lunch with two guests. After they left, Dee made it clear that she wanted to shop for clothes. I took her to a small women's clothing store in Payson. "No! I want the Valley" (Phoenix metropolitan area), she insisted. So given her good mood, I decided to try it. She was patient on the way down and we shopped in several stores, buying a pullover blouse at Macy's and several items at Talbot's. She was in shopper's heaven. She even allowed me to stop at the PGA store to get new grips for my golf clubs before we had dinner at a Chinese restaurant, followed by ice cream next door and the best coffee ever to go. She stayed awake all the way home and was soon in bed asleep.

I sent the following email to our youngest son because of his concern for his children's safety:

[Son],

Dee is doing much better now that she is off all medication. I doubt there will be any problem with your family staying in the downstairs rooms, because we spend nearly all of our time upstairs. However, we would welcome you here earlier to scope out the situation. You could be a big help to me if I still have ALTCS or tax return information to assemble by taking Dee on walks, to get groceries, or working together with her on picture albums. You could come up Monday and Tuesday and sleep over two nights. You could also join me at the men's breakfast Bible study on Wednesday morning and maybe equally important at the Alzheimer's support group on Wednesday afternoon, 1:30 p.m. to 3:30 p.m. while [our lady friend] is in the house doing housework and looking after Dee. If [your wife] and the children could come up before lunch they could spend time with Dee while we are gone and prepare a vegetarian meal for dinner.

Dee responds well in social environments, especially with people she loves and children in particular, so I doubt there will be any problems. However, she typically eats lunch by 11:30 a.m. and dinner by 5 p.m. This later time is because of her "sundowning." If I wait until later she can get quite upset. Hunger and anger go together. Routine is important. This will also apply on Saturday for the reunion events. I will give her snacks before the lunch to help tide her over until noon and she and I will likely leave the pizza dinner by 6 p.m. to get her to bed.

The most important thing with Dee is to keep her occupied doing something, just watching or listening is okay, all the time she is awake. She needs help with everything. I help her get dressed and go to the bathroom where I help her wipe and dispose of the paper in the toilet, and wash her up if necessary. I have to set the table, although if given the tableware she can sometimes get it on the place mats. She can eat by herself if I make sure she has her apron on and is sitting near the table. I also have to cut up meat (no problem while you are here) or she will pick it up and eat it with her hands. Since being off medication she is much more likely to be pleasant during these times and willing to assist doing what she can.

I hope that this will continue through the time that your family is visiting. I think that some of the drugs were making her crazy. Without them she just lacks memory and verbal skills and is generally pleasant if kept busy, but is sometimes rather despondent owing to her lack of ability. I cannot say that I blame her.

Love,

Dad

SATURDAY, MARCH 15, 2014 ❧

The frequent bowel movements continued through Friday. However, Dee slept without urinating or dumping all through the night and woke up today completely dry. She went to the bathroom and had an early morning bowel movement and later went to the bathroom to urinate. She seemed to regain her ability to recognize when she needs to go. We went with friends to a potluck lunch and Dee did great. She was happy all day. I am so happy for days like this.

THURSDAY, MARCH 20, 2014 ❧

I took Dee into the shower with me this morning and washed her hair and body while she hit me several times, banged hard on the glass shower door, and said, "I hate you." She calmed down by lunchtime and seemed happy when a lady from church showed up, but she kept coming into the office to bother me while I tried to get ALTCS information together. When I told her to go back to the living room and entertain her guest, she slapped me hard on the head with her ring finger. I slapped her equally hard on the butt, to her wide-eyed surprise, and said firmly, "Never slap me again on my head. Get out of the office and take care of your guest." Then I closed and locked the door to the office. This is so damn frustrating!

SUNDAY, MARCH 23, 2014 ❧

The past few days Dee has had a serious problem with constipation. She had several signals for bowel movements but could not get them out. She no longer knows how to push with her stomach muscles so just sits for a very few minutes and gets up, only to repeat the process. I called the hospice nurse to get something to help Dee go, got the medication, and gave it to her disguised as decorations on ice cream. At about ten last night, after sleeping several hours, she came into the office and said, "See what I'm doing," as she pooped gobs and gobs on the rug and floor. I cleaned her up and got her back in bed with a diaper on and spent over an hour cleaning up. She had several smaller dumps and diaper changes in the night and morning.

TUESDAY, MARCH 25, 2014 ❧

Dee awoke today bright-eyed, loving, and cooperative. We went to yoga and she did well. Dee went shopping with two women from church after lunch to get new yoga pants and a blouse. She also purchased a yoga mat and a stylish white spring jacket. We invited one of the women and her husband to join us for our wedding anniversary dinner and had great fun from five thirty until nearly eight. Once home Dee agreed to let me get her clean before bed and is now fast asleep. It has been a wonderful fifty-third anniversary day.

MONDAY, MARCH 31, 2014 ❧

I only remember a few details from the previous week. Dee was very agitated on Wednesday, probably from too much excitement on our anniversary. A friend came over Thursday to witness me signing power of attorney documents with two women from the attorney's office. That afternoon the hospice social worker came to help with an interview by a social worker for the state to determine Dee's medical eligibility for ALTCS. Dee passed with flying colors by not remembering her own name, my name, the date, the year, the president, or anything else. Nevertheless, she insisted that she could take care of herself. I pointed out that Dee has lost continence almost completely. The interviewer had no doubt that Dee is a prime candidate for the ALTCS program.

SUNDAY, APRIL 5, 2014 ❧

Well, the first week of April has come and gone. It started out well with our youngest son arriving the afternoon of the thirty-first and spending lots of time with Dee looking over diaries of her childhood that he put together and picture albums from the past. This gave me time to prepare meals and get more of the ALTCS application done. Dee really enjoys having our son around. On April 1 we cleaned up the basement for the arrival of his family. On Wednesday, Dee did her usual activities with our helper while my son and I attended both the men's Bible study breakfast and afternoon Alzheimer's support group meeting. This upset Dee, but she forgot her anger when our daughter-in-law and the grandchildren arrived in the late afternoon. Dee was really positive through the end of the week as she helped purchase flowers and watched her daughter-in-law and granddaughter weed the garden and plant several potted plants and vegetable seeds.

On Friday evening, my birthday, our oldest son and his family arrived for dinner. It went well and lasted until late, with Dee in really good spirits. Saturday was equally successful when other relatives arrived. We went to the casino for a mini-reunion lunch to recognize my brother's eightieth birthday. Dee remembered and treated each relative with love and care. That evening we gathered at a hotel for a pizza dinner and a surprise birthday party for me. Dee wanted to leave immediately after finishing two slices of pizza but stayed on happily after a niece brought out a whole bunch of cupcakes with lighted candles to celebrate my birthday. I read the goofy cards aloud to everyone's laughter, and Dee forgot all about wanting to go home. Sunday morning the family attended church at eleven, during which Dee helped serve communion with assistance. She was radiantly beautiful in her deacon's robe and broke into tears of happiness as she helped serve communion to members of our family.

FRIDAY, APRIL 25, 2014 ?♥

Most of the weeks in April have gone well, with Dee off all medication. She has lost control of her urinary and bowel functions, but I insist on her wearing adult diapers and check on her regularly to make certain they are still on. If not, I put on another diaper and search for the one she threw away . . . someplace.

Dee has lost nearly all understanding of words. If I tell her to pull up her diaper it is likely to go down. Or she takes off her blouse. In church she sings beautifully and loudly in gibberish, no meaning at all to what she is singing. She cannot listen to the news or even listen to me read from the paper. She doesn't get any of it. She does enjoy watching tennis or golf, where she sees something happening.

I prepared and signed the deeds required to transfer our New Mexico property into my name only. I also changed other deeds to ensure that if I die first any remaining assets will go directly to our sons so Dee will never have enough assets to bump her off ALTCS. On Wednesday she joined me for an Alzheimer's support group presentation that lasted for over two hours. I think Dee would be a whole lot better off now if she had taken no drugs.

TUESDAY, MAY 13, 2014 ࿇

The hospice social worker informed me today that Dee no longer qualifies for hospice care because she has gained weight and is completely off medication. This upset me because I counted on their help. But the social worker said that they had no choice. It is in their licensing agreement with the state. So Dee and I are back on our own with help from several friends and part-time paid caregivers. Dee maintains her enthusiasm for social interaction, especially with her women friends from the church. They keep coming in twos for three hours about twice a week to take Dee out to lunch, to shop, and to a movie or some other activity. This works out well.

It helps a lot to have two women with her at a time so they can chitchat, laugh, and sing. Dee enjoys the interaction even though she cannot contribute. This gives me enough time to take a long walk, keep up with bills, and prepare the ALTCS application. I have hired a woman from a private for-profit service agency to come to our home three hours on Saturday mornings to prepare casseroles, hot dishes, cookies, cakes, and the like while I get stuff done around the house. I hope that all these helper ladies can meet ALTCS requirements so we will not have to start over with other qualified persons when the application is approved.

THURSDAY, JUNE 12, 2014 ࿇

The past month has been one of ups and downs. Dee's mood changes some days, sometimes minute to minute. She says she loves me, then hates me, wants me near, or wants me to go away. But she's not hitting or trying to hurt me physically. That is a welcome change. She begrudgingly lets me clean her bottom after bowel movements and replace her diapers after she soils them. She lets me wash her most nights but resists on other nights, especially when I try to clean her private parts. I don't blame her. It is the ultimate loss of self-control, privacy, and dignity to have someone do this, even one's husband.

Last Sunday the pastor asked us in church to think about what defines us, about who we really are. I am glad he did not call on me to answer because I did not know. After thinking about it for a couple of days, I concluded that I am a housewife. I also realize now how much Dee enabled me in my professional pursuits. She was my best friend and supporter in everything I did and accomplished professionally. Now her requirements force me to be another person. Dee, of course, has lost everything that defined her. She is no longer the accomplished educator and minister nor the cheerful, supportive, willing, and loving spouse. She sometimes is cheerful and loving. She often is grumpy, moody, and unkind. She is like a baby experiencing her terrible twos.

Over the last several days Dee developed a new behavior. If she is unhappy for any reason, she sneaks downstairs and crawls onto the bed in one of the guest rooms. She's doing that now. I take advantage of this downtime to get work done and add to this epistle.

One day while taking a shower with me, Dee grabbed and twisted the handle on the shower door so hard that the tempered glass exploded, with glass landing all over the floor. I told a very frightened Dee to stand still while I put a towel over the glass on the rug outside the shower and held her hand as we stepped out. I dried her and myself and closed the door when we left the bathroom. I spent an hour or more cleaning up the mess and then ordered a replacement without a handle. A day or two later we got a flat tire in the Prius and discovered that the tires had to be replaced. Then the passenger window in the Tacoma decided to go all the way up but only halfway down. The service department at the Toyota dealership discovered a bent frame probably caused when Dee slammed the door really hard during one of her angry spells. The vinyl floor in the office is falling apart and must be fixed as soon as I get the filing cabinets emptied of outdated materials, some to shred, others to recycle. Two weeks ago the two-year-old washing machine quit. Sears could not get someone to fix it for five weeks, so I hired a local man to repair it. His repair lasted one wash cycle. After $170 for useless repairs,

I bought a new washer. So why all of this all at once? It sure taxes my ability to cope.

MONDAY, JUNE 23, 2014 ❧

Dee became so overstimulated during a potluck lunch on Sunday that she could not sit still and spilled everyone's drinks when she pushed on the table to get up. I finally got her to sit down and eat most of what was left on her plate, but only after she jumped up several more times for no apparent reason. I strained a rib muscle trying to pull her chair to the table.

I am now trying to get our taxes ready for 2013 after filing for an extension on the April deadline. There is very little time to do this and nothing can be left on the desk when Dee is around. Dee's mood is so variable—sometimes good, often bad—that I am really stressed.

WEDNESDAY, JULY 9, 2014 ❧

I cannot remember anything unusual about the past two weeks. Time flies and little gets done except watching after Dee. But usually this is okay. When she is happy her smile helps so much, but the seesaw continues. This morning Dee refused to shower. Actually, I think she did not want to undress in front of me because she does not recognize me. Eventually I got her undressed and into the shower while she kept saying, "I hate you!" I just took it and proceeded to wash her hair and body. She did not cooperate and, in fact, ran out of the shower wet. So I let her run around the house wet and nude while I finished my shower. I finished drying her after I dried myself.

We went to the painting class, where I helped her paint an abstract while trying to work on my own painting. Dee kept complaining and said she had to go home right now . . . after being in class for less than an hour. So I cleaned up the paints and brushes and told the instructor that we likely would not return, that I simply cannot paint when Dee is around. I let Dee know I was upset and she replied, "You hate me!" And for the first time I almost agreed.

"I am tired of your selfish complaining without any thought for my feelings. I have feelings too and don't appreciate your unthankful and hateful attitude toward me," I told her.

Dee seemed shocked and sad to hear me say this and said she was very sorry several times on the way home. I told her I accepted her apology and hoped she would be more thoughtful in the future.

As I type this, I have been reading it back to Dee, though I doubt anything will change. Sometimes she is nice and loving; other times she is mean, thoughtless, and hateful. That's our life! I am supposed to remain calm, thoughtful, and loving all the time. It's a hard slog!

SATURDAY, JULY 26, 2014 ❧

The last couple of weeks we had mostly good times, but also what could have been a hilarious home movie if someone had recorded it. I picked some Swiss chard from my garden one morning and cleaned it in the sink. Dee threw it in the garbage. I rescued and rewashed it and admonished her not to do this again, then left to do something while it dried. When I returned it was gone. This time I did not find it. This was only the beginning. After supper Dee wanted some blueberry pie with coffee ice cream on top, so I gave her some. While I refilled her glass of water, she picked up my plate with the fork hanging precariously over the edge.

"Put down the plate before the fork falls on the floor!" I shouted.

This startled her and she pushed the whole plate off the high counter onto the lower counter. Amazingly, everything stayed on the plate. As I returned to the counter to finish my pie and ice cream, Dee jumped up with half of her pie and ice cream still on her plate. I quietly asked her to please put it down. This time she threw the plate up in the air and it landed face down on the carpet, making a big mess. This really pissed me off and I let her know with angry words while I worked to clean the carpet before the blueberries stained it permanently. In retrospect it is pretty funny to imagine.

TUESDAY, AUGUST 5, 2014 ❧

Nearly a month has passed with no major changes in Dee's condition, but this past week brought a wonderful change for me. Our youngest son came to stay with us for a few days. We enjoyed good times on Tuesday and Wednesday, playing a lot of pool in the basement. Our son played for his mom and generally won, so Dee enjoyed her frequent victories. Then we packed for a brief trip to San Diego to see my sister and her children and grandchildren. Our son is so good, gentle, thoughtful, and loving with his mother. I am really proud of him. As I drove toward the town of Oceanside, our son played CDs with lots of rhythm. Dee loved it. She swayed, clapped, sang, and laughed with joy. We enjoyed delicious meals and times together with my sister and her family the following two days.

Back at home, Dee kept trying to recall my sister's name and wanted to see her again. I explained that we could not because of the distance, but she made it clear that she wanted to talk with her. So I called and put the phone on speaker while Dee talked happy gibberish to my sister and she replied as if she knew what Dee was saying. Finally, Dee said, "Bye," and went to bed.

THURSDAY, AUGUST 14, 2014 ❧

Dee seemed happy with me after lunch so I asked if she would now like to take a shower and wash her hair. She said yes, but then walked out of the house and over to a neighbor's house to ask if she could live with her instead of with me. Dee soon returned home but with the neighbor calling ahead to make certain I was home. I locked the two front doors behind Dee so she could not walk out again. This time Dee let me help her undress, and when we were both undressed and ready to shower, she said she loved me and snuggled her nude body against mine. What a surprise!

MONDAY, SEPTEMBER 1, 2014 ❧

Nothing too special developed from mid-August until almost September. Dee and I ate out with friends on the thirtieth, where I ordered an iced coffee to drink. It was bitter and acidic so I added lots of cream. Once home, I got Dee in bed and developed a stomachache that got worse every hour through the night, even though I took multiple Tums and anti-gas pills. I got very little sleep but decided to go to Sunday school and church anyway. About halfway through service the pain in my stomach became so severe that I had to go to the emergency room. I called a lady friend and, thankfully, she agreed to meet us at home and stay with Dee for the day and overnight if necessary.

I drove to the hospital's emergency entrance and received multiple tests as doctors tried to figure out the cause of my pain. This resulted in an overnight stay. Our lady friend asked another lady from our church to help her and they stayed overnight with Dee. But Dee wanted to be with me so they brought her to the hospital, where I reassured Dee that my condition was not serious. I had pancreatitis and would only be in the hospital overnight. She seemed satisfied and tired so the ladies took her home and put her to bed. Dee was extremely upset the next morning when I was not home so the ladies again brought her to see me. This seemed to calm her, but when they returned home she was still upset and slammed a picture album down on one lady's head. Dee wanted me home right now. She calmed down when I got home and remained calm all afternoon. Now I wonder how Dee could be cared for if I had to be in the hospital for a week or more. I certainly could not rely on volunteers.

WEDNESDAY, SEPTEMBER 17, 2014 ह९

We have had mostly good days since I returned home from the hospital, but Dee's mood swings have been wide and often. She hit me (not very hard) several times and was really mad when I insisted that she take a shower. She returned to her more normal, happier disposition after the shower, especially as we danced to music from the 1950s in the living room. She even hugged and kissed me while we danced (from the waist up because her legs no longer respond to her mental commands, if there are any). It was fun to dance with her.

A further progression of Dee's lack of leg coordination occurred in yoga class. Dee fell several times when trying to move from sitting or squatting positions to standing. Her legs simply did not respond. She was really embarrassed when the instructor had to help me lift her up. When I asked Dee if she wanted to go to yoga class this morning she said yes, but when we got there she refused to go into the room and made it clear that she was done with yoga. I told the instructor of Dee's decision. The lady was gracious but relieved and said she hoped to see us from time to time.

When we got home I tried to do my yoga exercises. Dee did not like this, so I turned the '50s music up in the living room. She went in there and swayed to the rhythmic music. I am now assembling an elliptical machine in the basement so I can get regular cardiovascular exercise. Slow walking a few hundred feet with Dee does not cut it, and I cannot leave her with the caregivers.

FRIDAY, SEPTEMBER 19, 2014 ❧

ALTCS approved Dee, and her new case manager met with us. She felt that fifteen hours of care and two hours of respite for me each week would work. I also hired a lady from a social service agency to help us every weekday afternoon with dinner preparation, feeding, and getting Dee ready for bed. However, the first time she tried to get Dee washed up before going to bed, Dee grabbed and pulled a whole chunk of hair out of her head. I thought for sure we would be sued.

I added more respite care for two hours on Tuesdays to have another lady on private pay help with Dee and clean the house. Having the two women with Dee at the same time works well. They are able to wash and style her hair, dance to '50s Hit Parade songs, and laugh and sing hymns. If they have a good time, Dee has a good time. I now have approximately thirty-three hours of caregiving each week . . . actually more than what I absolutely need. But getting Dee familiar and friendly with a variety of caregivers is important. I would like to leave her with caregivers seven or eight hours at a time this fall so I can go fishing or do something else that I enjoy.

TUESDAY, SEPTEMBER 30, 2014 ॐ

I had the same two caregivers come from noon to five thirty and two women from the church come from five thirty to eight thirty while I went on a short fishing trip with two men from the church. I had a splendid time with the guys and apparently the day went well for the women, but when I got home Dee was in bed with some of her daytime clothes on and a loaded diaper. They said she would not let them change or clean her. They were wise not to try.

THURSDAY, OCTOBER 2, 2014 ॐ

Wednesday morning Dee was in a good mood but stood up more than straight, leaning back at the waist. She fell against furniture and the walls several times and to the floor once. She also fell down half a flight of stairs into the eight-foot-tall sliding glass doors at the landing without hurting herself or breaking the glass. Dee woke up cranky and uncooperative this morning and still had the distinct lean to the back and side that made her unstable. She was still bent over backward and sideways and falling against furniture and walls in the afternoon and I could not get her to sit down while I got supper ready. It was nerve-racking. I could not get her to lean forward to feed herself or for me to feed her without dropping food all over the apron on her lap. She knocked her glass of water off the table trying to get up and generally made a mess of things.

I had a major problem trying to get her ready for bed. She could not stand up, back up to the toilet, or do anything to help me take off her clothes. I got her to lean forward against the sink long enough to wash her face, but she could not stand up to let me help her put on pajamas. Rather, she sank to the dressing room floor and laid out flat. She was limp as a wet washcloth and I could not get her up, so I went into the bedroom to get the bed ready. When I returned to the bathroom she was sitting on the floor. She allowed me to help her up and to finish putting on her pajamas. She was so weak and tired that I had to hold her up while getting her into bed.

FRIDAY, OCTOBER 3, 2014 ஐ
I called the doctor's office, trying to discover the cause of Dee's posture problems. The certified nurse practitioner said to come right over. We did, and after checking Dee's vital signs the nurse said the condition probably resulted from a combination of dehydration and Dee's unwillingness to drink to make up for it. She also thought the dumps could have left her very low on potassium, which could contribute to a lack of muscular control. However, when we returned home I discovered that Dee had gotten into the chocolate laxatives I had hidden on the top shelf in the pantry and eaten some of them like candy. I threw the remainder in the outside trash can. I never know what to expect next.

MONDAY, OCTOBER 13, 2014 ஐ
The days go by so quickly that it is hard to recall everything that happened this past week. I know it went from good to bad and back again, over and over. I had a wonderful time golfing today after leaving Dee in a good mood with the two caregivers. They took her to a funny movie, where they shared a big bucket of popcorn and soft drinks. They followed the movie with a big scoop of ice cream and spent all but seventeen cents of the forty dollars I gave them. I came home happy to a happy Dee, happy to see me. She willingly let me get her ready for bed and went to sleep soon after I tucked her in. Today helped me realize how lucky I was to have Dee as my wife for so many wonderful, love-filled years.

Our oldest son and his family visited today to see what they could do to make my life easier. Dee enjoyed looking at pictures with our son while I prepared breakfast. We stayed in the house while the cook baked cookies and a quiche and made beef stew. In the afternoon we took a long ride around town and went to the casino to see an art show. Dee could not stand the large crowd and wanted to leave immediately, so this activity lasted only a few minutes. After shopping, Dee watched her granddaughter play pool while I exercised on the elliptical machine.

SUNDAY, OCTOBER 19, 2014 ॐ

We sat together in church today and Dee behaved throughout the service. Our children noticed how enthusiastically she sang and wandered about, looking for people to greet with a hug. I warmed the quiche for lunch, but Dee refused to eat or drink anything. She would not let our son help her and became very agitated. She stamped around and threw a glass of water that shattered all over the floor in front of him. His wife and daughter tried to stay out of the way because of Dee's combativeness. They feared getting hit by something. Dee did not say goodbye when they left for New Mexico. I could tell that our son was hurt by her behavior, so I asked him to remember that this was not his mother. "It's Alzheimer's disease. Your mom cannot help herself." They left without Dee offering a goodbye to anyone, but with a better understanding of what she and I experience daily.

THURSDAY, OCTOBER 23, 2014 ॐ

This "journey to unknowing" is proving to be very convoluted, with some relatively good days, some bad days, and some really awful days. Dee gave the lady caregivers on Tuesday a lot of trouble when I ran errands. She stomped around the house unwilling to do anything with them, then slipped on a throw rug near the living room entry and fell so hard against the outside wall that she shattered the plastic cover on an electrical outlet next to the door. Fortunately she did not get hurt.

Dee fell off the side of a chair another day when she would not allow the caregivers to assist her. There must be a perceptual disconnect between what she sees and the command given by her mind to her legs. She looks at the chair but sits down on its right edge. That evening Dee quickly pushed away from the table and fell hard onto the falling chair, knocking off its upholstered seat. Her pajamas and diaper caught on an exposed screwhead that ripped them wide open, but Dee was not scratched. I gently pulled her to her feet and set the chair aside for repair. She lovingly hugged me and seemed to thank me for helping.

MONDAY, NOVEMBER 3, 2014 ॐ

When we went to our dentist today for a routine teeth cleaning, he discovered that Dee had an abscessed molar and said that the abscess might be the cause of her recent surly behavior. I think so, too, but cannot figure out how her tooth can hurt horribly one day and not the next. The dentist and I discussed doing a root canal but concluded that it could not be done successfully because Dee had clamped her teeth down hard on his hand and the dental hygienist's cleaning instruments several times. He suggested having a specialist in the Valley pull the tooth with Dee sedated. This idea did not thrill me because I wondered how much she would resist and how the sedation would affect her memory. But having no other real choice, I agreed.

WEDNESDAY, NOVEMBER 12, 2014 ॐ

Dee resisted about everything all day and threw the contents of a coffee milkshake at me after lunch. The shake went all over the dining room table, carpet, and me. Pissed, I flipped the shake material on my right hand at her face, missed completely, and splashed it on the wall behind her. Our lady helper entered the house just as I missed. She laughed at the situation, and Dee, seeing her laugh, responded with laughter. The lady cleaned up the floor and I cleaned off the wall while Dee stormed around the house bumping and hitting the furniture, walls, the lady, and me. She continued this behavior all afternoon with the two of us and with another caregiver when she came to help. Dee grabbed the caregiver's arm so hard I thought it might break. The lady screamed and I had to hit Dee's knuckles hard to make her let go. Later Dee bounced around the house with remarkable fury and eventually fell over and completely demolished a small end table in the living room. Fortunately, again, she was not hurt. It is amazing how many times she has fallen hard and gotten up without a scratch, bump, bruise, or broken bone. But she is wearing out the odds.

I am sure the abscessed tooth is giving her considerable pain and she needs relief. But never once has she placed her hand on her jaw or pointed out the nature of the problem. It has to be so painful and frustrating for her, and I cannot blame her for the bad behavior. Apparently, the abscess sends a signal to her brain, but the brain does not know where the signal came from.

THURSDAY, NOVEMBER 13, 2014 🖊

My life is now some kind of hell and Dee's is an even worse hell. Something has to give! Many people told me that the earlier you place your loved one in a memory care facility the better. Others say you must do this while you can still remember your loved one fondly, not wait until you hate him or her. Well, I already hate what she does during her angry times. But I remember very fondly the Dee I courted, married, and lived with happily for over fifty years. She was such a lovely person, accomplished professional, and wonderful, loving, caring wife and mother. I could not have asked for more. It is probably past time for me to see her off to a safer place where she can be comfortable and, if necessary, appropriately sedated to keep from hurting others and herself.

FRIDAY, NOVEMBER 14, 2014 🖊

We got up early and drove to Scottsdale for Dee's appointment with the dental surgeon. Dee behaved until we got to the surgeon's office and they asked us to wait. She could not wait. So I told the receptionist that we would walk around outside and to call us when the surgeon was ready. We walked around a long time and returned to ask the receptionist to have the surgeon hurry up. Dee could wait no longer. The receptionist said that the surgeon was ready and walked us back to the operating room. However, Dee would not let the surgeon and nurse get her on the operating table. He called for another nurse, but seeing their inability to accomplish the task I stepped in to help. Finally we had Dee on the reclining chair/table and they quickly administered anesthesia. Dee went out like a light and the surgeon asked me to leave while he extracted the tooth.

After only a few minutes the surgeon came out and said the tooth came out easily and that he had cleaned up the infected puss and covered the opening with sterile gauze. He gave me extra gauze to replace the bloody gauze in her mouth. However, Dee jerked out the gauze when she woke up and would not allow anyone to insert another piece. Still quite dizzy and apparently swallowing the oozing blood, she sat quietly and dozed off several times on the drive home.

SUNDAY, NOVEMBER 16, 2014 ᴓ
We got up this morning in time to shower, dress, and have breakfast before Sunday school and church. I chose not to try to protect Dee's clothes at a potluck lunch at the church because she had already eaten several chocolate chip cookies and wiped her hands on her clothes. I got her all the messy food she wanted. She ate it with her hands—with much of it landing on her slacks. When we got home, she looked in the mirror at her clothes with disgust and expressed her displeasure. She gladly agreed to change clothes and I, of course, changed her diaper at the same time.

Dee was hungry and became upset as I prepared dinner. She threw stuff around and refused to cooperate. She would not eat the soup nor drink the cider and wanted to go to bed at five but would not agree to undress or wash up. I persisted angrily and forcibly undressed her, put her in bed, shut the blinds, turned off the lights, and had dinner by myself. Dee came to the dining room crying her heart out as I finished. She was very sad. Inconsolable! I got her to sit on my lap and apologized for being so angry, but she continued to weep while she ate. Afterward, with her still sobbing, I put her into bed, feeling terrible about her broken heart. Apparently not all of Dee's behavior relates to the abscessed tooth. Some is from hunger and some is from my unkind behavior. I feel like a real jerk.

THURSDAY, NOVEMBER 20, 2014 ॐ

I researched memory care facilities in the Payson and Phoenix areas November 18 to 20. These facilities charge between $3,000 and $8,000 per month for Alzheimer's care private pay. Some contract with ALTCS, but others require two years of private pay and then allow the patient to continue on ALTCS. However, once a person is off ALTCS there is no guarantee that they can get back on, so the attorney and others advised me not to consider these facilities. I called ALTCS to see about getting more hours at home, but eighteen to twenty hours is the maximum each week for home care, and they will only place Dee in an ALTCS-approved facility when she needs full-time care.

I made a list of ALTCS-contracted facilities in Payson and will check out the ones I have not already visited. I am not optimistic about Dee getting good care in any of these facilities. Some are more like warehouses where patients sit in front of a TV set all day.

MONDAY, NOVEMBER 24, 2014 ॐ

I was surprised to find that two home care facilities Dee and I visited were quite nice and apparently well run. They were clean and the residents seemed happily engaged in various activities. The owners were pleasant and professional and the staff happily interacted with the patients. The larger one had ten beds, with one women's bed open and one woman on hospice care looking much like Dee's mom when the end neared. The smaller home had six beds. Five were for women and one for a man. They also had an open bed for a woman. The other bed in the room was in use by a woman on hospice care also looking like the end was near. This second home is an enlarged double-wide run by a young couple. Dee related well to both the wife and husband while sitting with them at the dining table. I could imagine Dee living in either of the homes, but I am not sure they can handle her surly behavior.

Dee and I visited the second home again to let them know of my interest to have her live there. We visited soon after I gave her .5 ml of lorazepam at lunch. I discussed this drug with the owner because of Dee's unsteadiness after taking it. She said that lorazepam does that to elderly people and she does not let her residents take it for fear of their falling. "The only persons that should take it are those unable to get up and move around," she said.

I decided to go to our doctor's office to discuss Dee's drugs. To my surprise and pleasure, the nurse practitioner immediately came to the waiting room to greet us and led us back to one of the examination rooms. She agreed with the owner of the second home and made a prescription for Zoloft, an antidepressant also used to treat anxiety. Dee had a low-grade fever and the nurse said we should get a urine sample to check for another urinary tract infection. The nurse used a catheter to get some fluid directly, with considerable resistance from Dee. While getting the sample the nurse noticed discharge in the area, making a urinary tract infection likely. She gave me prescriptions for a liquid antibiotic to address this condition. I have given Dee these drugs the past two days but she is still surly. I hope that curing the infection will calm her down.

While I write this Dee is finally in bed asleep. She got up earlier and sat on my lap with a nice smile and I gave her a big hug, only to discover that she had leaked while in bed and that the back of her pajamas, and now my pants, were soaked. So I changed her pajamas, my pants, and the bottom sheet on her bed after cleaning the mattress protector. Par for the course!

I told the nurse about my search for memory care facilities and my pleasant surprise at finding two small homes in the Payson area that seem to do a good job. She suggested trying one for a two-week period to see how Dee gets along. I think this is a good idea, but because of the experience we had at the nursing home, I am afraid that Dee will not do well anyplace. I am inclined toward trying the smaller one because of the presence of the young couple, both of whom are friendly, healthy, and strong. It can take two strong people to handle Dee when she does not want to cooperate.

I also want to visit two or three of the larger memory care facilities in the Valley for comparison purposes. But I am strongly inclined to try the local facilities so I can visit Dee regularly without having to spend four hours on the road each time I see her. This way I can pick her up and go to church on Sundays and to the movies, bowling, golfing, or just driving around on other days. It could become more like dating again . . . rather than being the primary caregiver, feeding her and cleaning up her messes. This sounds good to me. Will it be good for Dee? I do not know.

WEDNESDAY, NOVEMBER 26, 2014 ᷀❧

Dee responded well to the antibiotics for her urinary tract infection and enjoyed Sunday school, church, lunch with friends, and watching TV movies on Sunday afternoon. On Monday, two ladies from the church took Dee out for lunch and to a movie while I continued to get information on memory care facilities in the Valley. Tuesday was simply horrid, with completely uncontrollable behavior for reasons unknown to me. Today we revisited both assisted living homes in the Payson area to talk more about Dee's capabilities and behavior and to ask questions about how they would care for her. I learned a lot about each facility and the hesitancy of the first owner to take Dee. This was not the case for the second, smaller facility, where the owner seemed sure that Dee would do well in their home. She said that her approach is to stay positive and back off from negative behavior, coming back later when the patient is more receptive. This does work for Dee sometimes. The problems come when I am tired or want to finish something like cooking, cleaning, writing checks, keeping books, etc., etc.

I arranged for Dee to begin her stay at the smaller home on December 8 to allow me time to finish giving her the antibiotics for her urinary tract infection, get her stabilized with the Zoloft, have the certified nurse practitioner write an admission/transfer order, and get Dee a tuberculosis test with results. The lady agreed to this arrangement, provided I give her a nonrefundable $500 deposit to cover Dee's costs in case ALTCS does not pay in a timely manner . . . something she expected would happen. I agreed to this and took her a check.

So a new phase of our lives is beginning. Dee and I will no longer be living together if the respite care works out. I like the idea of her living nearby where I can pick her up each Sunday to take her to Sunday school, church, and to lunch with friends before returning her to the assisted living home. I like the idea of seeing her during the week without driving a long way to do it. I definitely will not miss getting her ready for bed. I will miss even less cleaning up after her bowel movements.

THURSDAY, NOVEMBER 27, 2014 ❧

I must say that I am thankful this Thanksgiving that our living situation will change. I am completely burnt out—*fried*, as one of our lady caregivers observed. I look forward to a new life where I can once again enjoy reading and writing books, skiing, fishing, hunting, and even playing eighteen holes of golf. I am looking forward to traveling to attend events, evening plays, and more in Phoenix and Tucson. I want to travel to see our children, grandchildren, other relatives, and friends. I want to travel to exotic places still on my wish list. I want to do watercolors without having to take the paint set and paintings down for fear that Dee will mess them up in some way. I want to breathe again!

TUESDAY, DECEMBER 2, 2014 ❧

This morning started off poorly, with Dee refusing to get out of bed and not wanting to get dressed. She had a bowel movement in her diaper that got on her legs and pajamas, and after cleaning her bottom I struggled to get her into the shower to wash off her lower body. She had another partial dump before breakfast that I cleaned up, but with her hitting me on the head and trying to escape. I decided that she was clean enough to go to the doctor's appointment, but when Dee got out of the car at his office, I smelled something familiar. I put her clean diapers and a washcloth in a plastic bag and took her into the doctor's restroom, hoping to change her without getting poop on her clothes, the floor, or me. She resisted and hit me on the head at least ten times, pinched me hard on both arms, and tried to stomp on my feet, but after a couple of ear-piercing screams she was reasonably clean. I could not say the same for the restroom. I wiped the toilet seat and the floor with the washcloth and towel but told staff that the room needed proper cleaning before anyone else used it. Fortunately the nurse came in at that moment and took Dee to the examination room to administer the TB test and make prescriptions for assisted living and stronger medication.

FRIDAY, DECEMBER 5, 2014 ॐ

The last three days have had their ups and downs. I managed to give Dee 3 ml of Zoloft before she went to bed the first evening, 4 ml the second, and most of 5 ml tonight before she spit out the last three sips of orange juice. During the day she remained mellow, even nice and loving at times. She held my hand for a while when I went to bed last night.

Dee fell in the garage Wednesday and over the hamper in the bedroom later that evening. I suspect that her unsteadiness relates to the increased dosage of Zoloft.

I hope and pray that the owners and other caregivers at the assisted living home in Star Valley can handle Dee, but frankly, I expect them to tell me to come get her because of her combativeness. I hope the next two nights of 5 ml of Zoloft will mellow Dee enough to allow them to change her into pajamas midafternoon without too much difficulty. Dee's behavior at the nursing home when I was supposed to get five days of respite last spring leaves me with trepidation that there will be a repeat. If I have to pick her up before the first five days are over, I will be unable to check out other facilities in the Valley and have no caregivers lined up to help when she comes home. I do not look forward to this. I am really tired of the daily battles . . . so I had better get to bed. Tomorrow will be a big day of preparation for Dee's move to assisted living.

SATURDAY, DECEMBER 6, 2014 ❧

I awoke this morning at five thirty to a loud thud and Dee's scream of pain when she fell out of bed. When I got the lights on and around the bed to her, she was trying to get up with her nose bleeding on the floor. I helped her stand and took her into the bathroom to wash the blood off her hands and face, then tried to comfort her while dabbing the blood until it stopped. She has a noticeable bruise on the right side of her nose. Maybe she tried to get out of bed with her legs and arms caught in the blankets, causing her to fall face first. We'll never know because Dee cannot tell me, even if she could remember. It is so sad. As soon as her nose quit bleeding, I took a wet washcloth and did my best to remove the blood on the carpet before it dried and set in.

Dee apparently had a bowel movement before or during the event because it filled her diaper. She cooperated with me as I tried to clean her bottom, but the poop was all over the inner part of her legs, so I decided to clean her properly in the shower. She cooperated and I did a thorough job cleaning, drying, and getting her dressed for a United Methodist women's brunch. I went back into the shower to wash up while she stood around passively.

I spoon-fed Dee the breakfast cereal this morning because she could not figure out how to do it. She then wandered around while I finished my breakfast. She had several outbursts of loud gibberish during and after breakfast while I made the beds and folded laundry. I also collected used paper products and recyclable plastics and metals with Dee tagging along. We let the cook in and I took the recycling to the dumpsters before a lady from church picked up Dee to go to the brunch. I also typed some instructions on caring for Dee to give to the owners of the assisted living home in Star Valley.

Dee came back from the brunch happy to have been out with her lady friends because they always treat her very nicely. I marked and packed a week's worth of clothing, diapers, and other items in her absence. Then we went grocery shopping for food and drink items to ease Dee's transition to the assisted living home's food and beverages. Dee was pretty mellow through the afternoon and evening as I prepared her for dinner and bedtime.

SUNDAY, DECEMBER 7, 2014 ❧

This was a nice warm and sunny day. Dee had a bowel movement just before Sunday school so we missed the first half while I cleaned her up. Greeting friends and church went well as usual. Then we hurried home for lunch and a trip to the golf course. This also went well. When we got home, I washed our hands and we had dinner before attending a Christmas rock concert at our church in the early evening. Dee listened intently through the whole event. I found it much too noisy. When we got home, Dee got into her pajamas and went straight to bed. This really nice day with Dee makes me think that the increased dosage of Zoloft is working.

MONDAY, DECEMBER 8, 2014 ❧

The day started well with our usual breakfast routine and last-minute packing before heading to the assisted living home. The woman owner met us at the door with her friendly smile. We took the suitcase to Dee's room and got everything in order for her stay. It became clear then that Dee did not like what she saw going on, so we sat and talked for a while with the co-owner in the living room. I could see Dee getting agitated because of hunger, so I asked and they prepared some soup for her. They sat her at a table with several other residents to eat the soup. At the owner's suggestion, I slipped out while Dee ate, in hopes of avoiding a scene.

I called later and they informed me that when Dee discovered I had left, she became agitated and would not sit down. Rather, she paced wildly from one end of the home to the other looking for a way to escape. She did this nonstop for several hours, drinking nothing, grabbing and gobbling down a few food items as she went by the table, and not letting anyone do anything for or to her. Finally she collapsed on the couch looking angry and just sat there. The owner eventually got her diaper changed and took Dee into the bedroom, where she immediately fell asleep.

They called me to sign a paper allowing them to video monitor Dee through the night to keep her and her roommate safe. I drove to the facility and signed the necessary papers. The owner still hoped that Tuesday would be an easier day but suggested that I consider having Dee go into a hospital's behavioral program to get her mood stabilized. I looked up the hospital's program on the Internet and it seemed like a good idea. In the morning, I called two memory care facilities in the Valley to see if they would care for a person like Dee. Both said they would not, that she had to be stabilized first. They agreed that stabilization at the hospital would be a good option.

TUESDAY, DECEMBER 9, 2014 ᥅❧

I waited until ten this morning to call the assisted living home to see if Dee's behavior had improved. It had not. Dee would not allow them to put on her clothes, nor would she eat or drink anything. She was scared, anxious, and angry. The owner said they could not handle her. Dee had thrown stuff around, knocked over the Christmas tree, and hit another resident while storming around the small home. The lady said that Dee had to be on medication to control her emotions and until that was done it would not be safe to have her at their home or any other facility. So the experiment lasted one day. I called the hospital and discovered that they could admit her the next day.

I made preparations to pick up Dee and take her to the hospital the following day, then drove to the home and looked through the door window to see Dee sitting on the living room couch, looking angry and tired in a room littered with adult diapers, pillows, and other items she had thrown on the floor. Dee ran to me and gave me a big hug and several kisses when I entered the room, her mood changing instantly.

The staff helped us carry Dee's belongings to the car, with the owner reiterating the necessity of medication to control Dee's behavior. Dee remained happy the rest of the day at home, almost like the Dee I have loved these many years. She consumed her soup like she had eaten nothing for days, which was nearly true, and gave no resistance to my washing her for dinner and bed. But I was convinced that she had to be stabilized. I emailed our children and my siblings of my decision but went to bed uneasy about it and did not sleep well.

WEDNESDAY, DECEMBER 10, 2014 ॐ

Dee awoke with her big, beautiful smile and radiated happiness as we followed our usual breakfast routine. She ate half of a large Gala apple and all of her cereal and drank all of her juice. I decided that I could not take her to the hospital just before Christmas with the distinct possibility that she would still be there when our children and grandchildren came at the end of the month. I visualized a very placid Deanna without her winning smile and sparkling eyes who could not remember me or anyone else. It was too sad to contemplate. I decided to keep Dee at home until our children came after Christmas and to have them help me make decisions.

THURSDAY, DECEMBER 11, 2014 ॐ

This day also went well while I set up the tree with lights. Dee assisted by taking out ornaments for me to put on the tree. One of our paid caregivers came at eleven and helped us finish decorating the tree. In the afternoon I put up the outside lights on the porch and on the Douglas fir in the yard. Dee wandered in and out of the house watching and stayed in a very good mood. This was true even when she tripped and fell hard on the terrace, landing on both knees and one elbow. She got up laughing. I knew it had to hurt because of the sound of bone hitting concrete, but she showed no signs of pain.

By the time we finished, Dee's sundowning had set in and she was not willing to eat dinner or clean up to go to bed. She grabbed my clothes and wrists, pinched my arms and chest, and did everything she could to resist taking off her clothes. I slapped her hand more than a few times to make her release a piece of clothing, or clenched it hard with my other hand to make her let go. I could not control my temper and eventually just latched onto both of her wrists with my right hand, turned on the lavatory water, put soap on the washcloth, and washed and rinsed her face and body with my left hand. She jerked and pushed and did everything to resist while I angrily got her ready for bed. It was a bad scene.

Our youngest son called while all this was going on and I simply said to him, "I'll call you later." I did and told him of my hopes and now my angst about how to deal with Dee.

FRIDAY, DECEMBER 12, 2014 ᴥ

This day went much better after an awful night during which Dee kept me awake jabbering incessantly and getting out of bed. She may have had nightmares relating to the difficult times before she went to bed. At about five twenty in the morning she started jabbering again, trying to tell me something important as she fell out of bed onto her face, with her legs and one arm caught in the blankets. The fall left a big bruise on the bone under her right eye. It remained red all day but at least so far has not resulted in a black eye.

Dee was very compliant as I got her dressed for the day and had breakfast. Afterward we went to the college for our painting class, only to find school out for the holidays. We then went grocery shopping, where Dee helped select some foods as we went up and down the various aisles. This was unusual because for the past several months she has been very passive at the grocery store, just walking along with me. We did various errands during the afternoon and were home by four to get her ready for dinner and bed. Here again she cooperated, even as I cleaned up a major bowel movement. I thought to myself that perhaps we could carry on this way indefinitely if I just stick to a rigid schedule . . . and pay attention to her needs at all times.

SATURDAY, DECEMBER 20, 2014 ∂❧

The past few days went by like a whirlwind as we began preparations for Christmas and visits from our children and their families. Dee had the same mood swings as before: sometimes happy, even cheerful; other times dower and combative. She seems to have less and less leg strength for getting up from a seated position and getting her right leg into the car. I watch carefully to make sure she does not slam the door on her foot and have intervened just in time on several occasions. It's easier for me if I pay attention to her all the time. This means that the only time to get other things done is after she is in bed and asleep. However, while she is often in bed by seven, she is up repeatedly until about nine, before she is down for good. Consequently, like tonight, I will not go to bed before eleven in order to get needed chores done . . . writing checks, balancing books, replying to emails, and the like.

After the first application of the calming gel on Tuesday, when I went to the Valley to check out memory care facilities, Dee apparently hit a new caregiver very hard on her shoulder. The caregiver went to urgent care because of nerve pain and told her supervisor that she would not come back to care for Dee. I wonder if we are in for a lawsuit. Now, only the private pay caregiver and one good friend seem able to manage Dee safely when I am away. The other caregivers make valiant efforts, but I think Dee senses their fear and bullies them. It requires at least two caregivers to change her diaper or to wash her for bedtime. I do not ask them to clean up after bowel movements because I know how difficult Dee can be. I do this, but it takes all of my strength to hold onto her with one hand and clean with the other. It is not fun for either of us.

The nurse practitioner took Dee off the Zoloft later in the week when I indicated that it seemed to make her nervous, even jittery at times, mumbling incomprehensible noises repeatedly at a very fast clip. The nurse said to use Thorazine gel on her arms or legs twice a day to try to reduce the anxiety. This has a peculiar effect, making Dee anxious and aggressive the first couple of hours, then mellow for a few hours. Today Dee stayed mellow until bedtime. I really wonder if any medications help her. Can the psychiatrists at the hospital figure it out? I hope so!

This evening as we watched TV Dee became happy, snuggled up, and told me how much she loves me . . . rather clearly in English. At times like this, when she behaves like the wonderful wife of the first fifty-two years of our marriage, my heart just aches to think about her being heavily medicated to keep her under control in an assisted living environment. At other times I can hardly wait to get her out of the house to regain some semblance of a life of my own. It is a terrible quandary about which I must make a decision soon, thankfully with the assistance of our children and their wives.

TUESDAY, DECEMBER 23, 2014 ୬♥

I had the two caregivers come at nine this morning so I could drive to the Valley to meet my younger son to check out three memory care facilities and the hospital's psychiatric ward with him. We stopped first at a very large multiservice health care facility in central Chandler. The dementia care's cleanliness impressed us, but the lack of access to an exterior area, long dark hallways, and passive behavior of all of the residents concerned us. We then visited the hospital, where the intake officer at the psychiatric ward impressed us with their approach. She said that admission would take only a day or two when space is available. She would not predict Dee's state of awareness when dismissed from the hospital. "Most patients maintain a near normal state of functioning without the belligerent behavior," she said. I hope this is true.

We also visited a large retirement center in Phoenix with a memory care facility on the fifth floor of a high-rise building. The quality of the staff and the activity level of the patients in memory care impressed us. However, the unit smelled old and needed refurbishing. I liked it better than the first facility because of its focus on individualized treatment and the apparent happiness of the staff and patients. But I still feel that the two small houses in Payson would be better with Dee's improved behavior.

We visited a memory care facility in north Phoenix last and liked the concept of seven identical twelve-person cottages located around an outdoor courtyard, where residents could roam freely in a secure environment. We also liked how they place new admissions with residents of similar capability and gradually move them to other cottages as their abilities change. The light-filled, clean, and well-organized units have been refurbished with new surfaces, furnishings, and very attractive colors and paintings on the walls. The staff seemed enthusiastic and professional. The residents also appeared to be happy with their care. I think Dee would do well there. The big drawback, of course, is its distance from Payson, a good hour and a half drive each way. However, I could drive down in the morning and take Dee to lunch, then out for some afternoon activity, before returning home in the late afternoon. Or I could stay overnight and pick up Dee early and drive back to Payson for church and lunch out with friends, then return her to the facility. I definitely feel that Dee would have the best quality of life in this facility.

Everyone I know and the ones we met on the trip, without exception, say it is past time for me to make a change. It is not good for either Dee or me to continue as we have for the past couple of years. I also think it will be best for both of us, but my heart yearns to have her remain with me here in our home. I can hardly bear the thought of separation after nearly fifty-four years together. But everyone counters that this way I can interact with her as my wife and loved one, not simply as her twenty-four-hour-a-day caregiver. This appeals to me.

WEDNESDAY, DECEMBER 24, 2014 ॐ

Dee and I had a very pleasant day together this Christmas Eve after a rocky start when she woke me at five thirty and kept pestering me until we got up at six thirty. But then she had her morning bowel movement sitting on the toilet, so I had very little cleanup to do. Yes! She did a lot of pacing up and down the hall in the morning while I did some follow-up calls, but since then her manner has been fairly mellow, including while we changed diapers and washed up for bedtime. We went to the movie *Annie* in the afternoon, after which she told me she loved me several times. I assured her that I felt the same way about her with several tender loving kisses. We also went out for a pizza dinner. I enjoyed being with her.

THURSDAY, DECEMBER 25, 2014 ৯৶
This Christmas Day also went well, with bowel movements over in the morning and Christmas dinner with good friends from the church at our home at lunchtime, but with them bringing all of the food. The friends stayed for about two hours and left when it became obvious that Dee was getting restless. We tried to go grocery shopping after dinner but even Walmart was closed. So we just drove around looking at Christmas lights before coming home and getting Dee ready for supper and bed. It was a pleasant if not memorable Christmas.

FRIDAY, DECEMBER 26, 2014 ৯৶
Today was special because both of our sons' families arrived to spend the weekend with us. Dee recognized our youngest son immediately and ran into his arms, kissed him repeatedly, and babbled about her affection for him. Her quick and genuine response surprised me. She then hugged and welcomed his wife and children. Our son immediately took Dee into his hands . . . but soon found out how difficult she can be.

Our oldest son and his family did not arrive until about eight thirty and wolfed down the stew, cookies, and ice cream that I prepared. Dee woke up and came to the living room to welcome them. I helped her back to bed at about nine thirty, after which our sons and I talked until after eleven about best options for Dee. We were divided a bit between placing her in an assisted living home in Payson and in a larger memory care facility in the Valley, but we agreed about getting her stabilized at the hospital's behavioral health unit, even though I had a nagging feeling that it would not work as intended given Dee's previous responses to medication.

I was really tired and went to bed without washing up, knowing that Dee would wake up during the night or very early in the morning. When I finally got to bed, Dee began muttering and swinging her arms around wildly. I had to grab her arms to keep them still. She resisted but I persisted until she finally relaxed. It seems like she has gotten back the demons from last winter when she was heavily medicated.

SATURDAY, DECEMBER 27, 2014 ❧

Sure enough, Dee awoke early this morning. By nine I had gotten her dressed and had everything set for breakfast for twelve people. After breakfast we sat near the Christmas tree in the living room while our youngest grandson delivered presents. Dee seemed content watching while I opened our presents, and she laughed when others laughed. Then the children and grandchildren opened their presents from us. We gave everyone gift cards to local stores with instructions to buy something they could make up a tall tale about later in the afternoon. The boys went to Big 5 Sporting Goods. The girls went to Rue 21. The rest of us went to Walmart. I hoped that buying gifts together would be a time of bonding for our sons' two families because they rarely see each other.

I grilled hamburgers and veggie burgers on the porch for lunch while the ladies set out the rest of the meal. Dee enjoyed watching the activity. She made a small mess on her apron while wolfing down the hamburger but enjoyed all the fun and laughter.

A moving moment came after most of us told some goofy story about our presents. Dee suddenly stood up and began to speak—mostly in gibberish but very emotionally—about her family. She motioned to each of us at various times and repeated words like "love" and "family" often as tears of happiness came to her eyes . . . and to ours as well. She could not make up some silly story about her gifts, but she could express how happy it made her to have her whole family together. It was clear to me how Dee, her essence, is still here. Her feelings and emotions are as strong as ever. Dee is still the wonderful, caring, loving person at her inner core. By early evening Dee was hungry so we had a light supper and I got her ready for bed. She went to sleep immediately but as usual got up several times before finally settling down for the night. She was clearly happy during this Christmas celebration with her family. I will always cherish that moment of clarity as Dee expressed her love for family.

SUNDAY, DECEMBER 28, 2014 ❧

Dee woke up early as usual but would not take a shower. I took mine and began to get dressed when she came back into the bathroom and agreed to shower. This went well, along with dressing her for the day. We all went to church and I had fun introducing everyone to the congregation, referring to our family members as "God sightings," the new pastor's terminology. After church we drove about fifteen miles to the Creekside Inn for lunch. Dee ate her cheeseburger quickly without a major spill, but when finished she wanted to return home immediately. So lunch broke up quickly, with our older son's family driving on to New Mexico and our youngest son's family returning home with us to watch football and chat. Dee was in bed by seven and only got up twice before settling down for the night.

MONDAY, DECEMBER 29, 2014 ❧

Dee woke up during the night a couple of times with wet diapers so I got up to change them. The third time she started swinging her arms, trying to wake me up. She'd had a dump. So I got up, changed her, and put her back in bed. I acted like I was also going back to bed but stayed up and did yoga because it was already six in the morning and I was unlikely to get back to sleep.

I contacted the hospital later in the morning to see if we could get Dee into the psychiatric ward for stabilization while my younger son could assist me. They were not certain at that point but said they would call me in the late morning or early afternoon if an opening occurred. I waited for a call all morning but none came. I called again after lunch and they said someone would call soon. At about three a lady called and said to come right away. I told them it would take us at least two hours to drive to the hospital from Payson and suggested that it was a bit late in the day. However, the lady insisted that we come as soon as possible. So I put the already prepared suitcase in the front seat of the car and had our son sit in the back with Dee. His wife and the children returned to her parents' home in Tempe in their car.

Our son brought three Hit Parade CDs along to play on the way down. Dee liked this and sang along on the familiar tunes. We got to the hospital about five thirty, where a nurse told us that we had arrived too late for processing by the staff currently on duty because it takes about three hours and the shifts change at seven. She said we would have to wait for the next shift to check in Dee. This disgusted us, but we could do nothing about it. Dee became increasingly agitated and wanted to go home. Instead, I decided that we should all go to the cafeteria and have dinner. This took about an hour. With time still on our hands, we bundled Dee up in all of the sweaters, jackets, and gloves we could find in the car and walked around the parking lot and grass areas surrounding the hospital, holding Dee's hands, for another half hour. Dee insisted that we return home. She was sleepy and wanted to go to bed. We listened but ignored her wishes. With time still on our hands, we went back to the main lobby and watched a bowl game for a short while. Dee did not like this so we took the elevator to the fifth floor to see if they were ready. They said they were just about ready and took us to a small room in the behavioral care wing to wait.

We waited another hour before a very obese and friendly paramedic came in. He took Dee's vital signs and went through a lot of paperwork. Dee gave him a scolding look, pointing at his big belly. My son and I apologized but he laughed and said it happens all the time and that he is trying to lose weight. This did not deter Dee from looking in disgust at his fat belly. Oh well.

Later a nurse came in to help us fill out and sign still other forms. Dee got more and more agitated as we did this. She was tired and wanted to go home to bed. I tried to explain to her that home was two hours away and that she would have to stay in the hospital for evaluation because she kept hurting people, including me, and needed to be stabilized. My explanation did not mollify her. She wanted to leave now. Finally a young, pretty Hispanic tech with a ready smile came in and we discussed next steps. The friendly paramedic and the young tech attempted to take Dee to her room but she resisted fiercely.

The nurse on floor duty came in and said that my son and I should vanish so they could get their job done. We started to leave, but Dee jerked loose and came running around the corner toward us with them in hot pursuit. Dee charged into my arms, where I told her, "I love you. You must stay with these people because they will help you get over your anger, hitting, and pinching problems." I said this earnestly and Dee seemed to understand. We hugged and kissed and she turned around and let them take her to her room.

My son and I left after completing more paperwork for the nurse. By then it was eleven thirty, several hours past Dee's normal bedtime . . . and ours as well. Our son had called his wife and her mother earlier to tell them that he and I would stay in a hotel overnight so as not to bother anyone if it got really late. We drove to Tempe and stayed in a hotel by the freeway.

TUESDAY, DECEMBER 30, 2014 ᴁ

After a short night's sleep, we drove to our daughter-in-law's parents' home and shared our story with them. I then drove to the memory care facility in northern Phoenix that my son and I liked to give them a $500 deposit and take care of paperwork. I met the owner of the facility and was as impressed with him as I was with the rest of the staff and facilities.

While there, I got a call from the psychiatrist at the hospital, who asked me many questions about Dee. I liked his thoroughness. He mentioned that I would have a conference with him, the nurse, and the social worker the following Tuesday to agree on a treatment plan. We could not meet on New Year's Day because some staff would be unavailable. His nurse called me later to get permission to have Dee take Aricept for Alzheimer's and another medication to help her sleep. I said yes to two different nurses to allow them to do this. I asked the first nurse how Dee was doing and she said very well. She stated that Dee had someone with her at all times and had slept for five hours. She had cooperated with the tech while taking off her pajamas, taking a shower, putting on a diaper, and dressing in the morning.

They did not keep any of the clothes I packed, so I assumed that Dee had on a light nightgown like I saw on the other patients in the ward. As we spoke, the nurse indicated that Dee was walking calmly in the hall with an aide and had been calm all morning. This pleased me and I happily called our sons and others about the good news. I was really hungry so I went to a resort hotel for lunch and played nine holes of golf. Then I met two friends from Payson at a restaurant in Fountain Hills before driving home, where I went to bed and slept for over nine hours.

WEDNESDAY, DECEMBER 31, 2014 ᐜ

I awoke this morning feeling really crummy and guilty about leaving Dee at the hospital. I ate at home because I did not feel like going to the men's Bible study breakfast. When I called the nurse at about ten, she indicated that Dee had resisted changing her diaper and cleaning up and refused to eat breakfast or take her pills. The nurse said that Dee responded better when they changed from the male night tech to the female day tech so they will try to follow up with women for all shifts. She asked me to approve a medication that could be injected into Dee's arm if she continued to reject pills. A second nurse came on the phone to confirm my approval. I felt terrible after the call, knowing that I left the love of my life in the hands of strangers on New Year's Eve. We had celebrated every New Year's Eve together since 1960. Now I am alone in the big house I designed to share with Dee during our retirement. Dee is undoubtedly confused by my absence and probably very sad as well in the hospital environment.

During the day I kept busy catching up, providing information to the care facility, and warming up a lunch for our caregiver friend and myself. She came to do laundry and clean the countertops as it began snowing heavily outside. It had snowed about nine inches by the time she left, leaving me alone in a house with limited groceries for supper. I drove to the church for a planned potluck only to find it canceled. I decided to eat at a new cafe where I could watch bowl games, feeling sorry for myself and worse for Dee as I sat alone eating and watching several games. It was the loneliest New Year's Eve of my life. I really missed Dee.

It does not feel right having Dee somewhere else, especially in the psychiatric ward of a hospital many miles away. My heart is broken even as my mind knows that our children, my brother and sister, and so many others are correct in saying that Dee must have her anxiety and hurtful behavior corrected so caregivers can handle her safely. It also must be done for her safety and for mine.

Our house is one big hazard, with too many objects to fall over or into, stairs to fall up and down, and glass windows and cabinet doors to break. Dee's anxiety and destructive behavior must be under control so others can care for her if I become unable to do it. Nevertheless, I am really sad and lonely and I miss my life partner. I hope with all my heart that the people at the hospital can come up with a treatment plan that will allow Dee to live happily in a memory care facility—that it will be such a good solution that I will be able to visit her several times each week and reclaim at least a dating relationship with this extraordinary woman as she declines further into the abyss of Alzheimer's disease.

Reflections on the Fourth Year ❧

I could not imagine our situation getting worse than at the end of 2013, but it could and did. Dee's on-again, off-again difficult behavior wore me down. The psychotic episodes that brought both fear to and hurtful behavior from Dee got worse. I did not fear for my life, but maybe I should have. Objects thrown or swung at me could have caused serious injury. If Dee had discovered a large knife in a kitchen drawer and gone after me, the result could have been even worse. If she had grabbed the steering wheel when I drove at seventy miles per hour toward Payson, she could have caused a rollover and we could have been seriously injured or killed. Dee took a number of spills over the year in our house, any one of which could have hurt her seriously, although none did. Her generally good physical health no doubt helped her avoid injury, but her string of urinary tract infections and abscessed tooth made our lives miserable.

I am truly sorry that I could not control my emotions better. I often got angry at Dee, even knowing that conditions related to Alzheimer's caused her misbehavior. Why couldn't I find something humorous in each encounter, smile at her lovingly, and even laugh with her to improve her mood and behavior? When two women at a time cared for Dee and laughed about something, Dee consistently laughed with them. She sensed that they were having fun and joined in. I wish I'd had the intestinal fortitude to do the same. But I didn't. I really wonder if insisting on completing the house project in New Mexico, especially when I worked with the bulldozer and expected Dee to stay on the porch and watch, caused her to develop a love/hate relationship with me, where previously it had been only a love relationship. Could her violent behavior be traced back to that period of time? I don't know, but I wonder.

I also wonder about the efficacy of any of the drugs used to treat Alzheimer's disease. Dee seemed to do better when I took her off the drugs. This was true for both Aricept and Namenda. It was true as well for the anxiety drugs. Was it because Dee never took drugs before she got

Alzheimer's and could not tolerate them, or that they do not do what they claim for people with this disease? The evidence with Dee certainly points toward ineffectiveness.

I feel even more strongly about the necessity of having family members nearby to support and relieve the caregiver. The times that our youngest son assisted with caregiving provided more respite for me than anything the paid helpers provided. I was, of course, also frustrated by Dee's unwillingness to accept care outside of our home so I could get away to care for myself. I wonder if our love-filled life prior to her getting Alzheimer's made such a separation so untenable for her. Would it have been easier if we did not love each other so much, or if we had entered an aging in place facility early in the course of her disease so that the transition from our living together in an apartment to her living in a memory care unit in the same facility would have been less drastic? I wonder.

The transition from continence to incontinence that began with Dee's brief negative experience in the care facility in Payson made caring for her at home much more difficult. It also resulted in episodes of urinary tract infection that must have been very painful and increased Dee's violent behavior. Adult diapers that work well for containing urine do not work well for loose bowels because they allow unwanted bacteria into the urinary tract. I don't know what to do about this. It leaves the caregiver between the proverbial rock and hard place.

Advice to Caregivers ॐ

1. If your loved one is incontinent and is a woman, be careful to keep feces out of the vagina and urinary tract. This is not easy when the person is wearing adult diapers or similar underwear to keep from soiling clothes or bedding. Be alert for the smell of feces and change the diaper before she sits down. I cleaned up feces at the toilet but when

possible moved my wife into the shower in the same room to remove the remaining feces with a handheld showerhead. It helps if there is a grab bar that your loved one can hold onto while you spray. Be sure to get the water temperature to a comfortable level first. Those with a bidet may be able to achieve the same result. But understand that your loved one may still get a urinary tract infection and be unable to tell you about it. My wife had at least two such episodes in two years and provided no clue to me about where her pain originated. If your loved one becomes unusually combative, have her checked ASAP for a urinary tract infection. It will save both of you a lot of pain.

2. We had a similar problem when my wife had an abscessed tooth. She never pointed to or rubbed her face or chin to indicate that it hurt, but her face contorted in pain during this time and she became very agitated and combative. We first checked for a urinary tract infection but the test was negative. We had no idea why she became so difficult until we went for a routine teeth cleaning and the x-ray showed an abscess. Leave no stone unturned to find the cause of difficult behavior or it will continue to your loved one's and your detriment. Apparently, Alzheimer's created a mental disconnect in my wife regarding the source of her pain. Maybe when the brain should be indicating pain in the jaw or groin it is felt only in the head as a severe headache. My wife had no ability to communicate where her pain originated.

3. I found taking a shower in the morning with my wife two or three times a week useful because I had little success trying to get her clean before bedtime. Sundowning is real. Before the shower, carefully select and set out clothes for your loved one to wear after the shower, if possible with his or her approval. Here again, I had my wife hold onto the grab bar in the shower to make it less likely for her to slip and fall. I also got the water to a comfortably warm temperature before using the handheld showerhead to spray and wash her legs and feet before cleaning the rest of her body. I usually could keep her in a

good mood in the shower if I waited till the end to wash her face and hair. She must have feared drowning or something similar because she would not allow anyone to wash her hair first or in a sink. Maybe this was unique to my wife. I do not know. I do know that she was happier after a shower if the room was warm and I dried her thoroughly before helping her dress.

4. I will emphasize, over and over, the importance of "love medicine." My wife needed to know that I loved her. Having family members and friends visit and help celebrate special occasions or just be around made Dee's life so much better. I did not ask them to do dirty work, but it would have been nice if paid help could have cleaned her up after bowel movements. Unfortunately Dee's combativeness made it impossible for them to do this. Maybe it would be possible for other people with Alzheimer's.

5. Taking my wife to church every Sunday, where she felt loved, was especially good love medicine. It will make your life better if you can find similar social activities. Friends talking, smiling, and laughing with my wife was much more productive than my anger. Try to show your love even when you feel hurt. (Easy to say but hard to do!)

6. At some point the caregiver must give up traveling with their loved one with Alzheimer's. Travel becomes too inconvenient if the person is incontinent and even dangerous if the person is agitated. Plan your activities within easy distance from home and toilet facilities. If you detect symptoms of anger, don't get behind the wheel. You will be an accident waiting to happen.

7. Try to find ways to take care of yourself while caring for your loved one. For me golf worked some of the time, bowling for a while, and the elliptical machine helped when I had to stay with Dee. You will need some way to stay in shape physically and mentally. I found that writing this diary was a way to let out my pent-up grief and anger at the end of the day so I could sleep at night. You will need some way to do this.

8. I am reluctant at this point to suggest giving any medication to your loved one. With Dee I saw no beneficial effect from Aricept or Namenda. If anything, they just prolong the disease. Anxiety medications seemed to create rather than alleviate mental problems. I wonder if all of the medications used with Alzheimer's patients are just a way to make more money for the pharmaceutical industry. I hope not.

5

Fifth Year
of the Journey

❧

Hospital Daily Excerpts ❧

THURSDAY, JANUARY 1, 2015 ❧

While watching bowl games and trying not to think about leaving my wife in a strange place, I started printing a bucket list of things to accomplish in the remaining years of my life. I filled out both sides of one 3 × 5 index card, then filled out another with things I need to accomplish in the near future. I tried without success not to think about Dee in the hospital, knowing it would be a very sad time for her.

FRIDAY, JANUARY 2, 2015 ❧

Still trying to keep my mind off Dee's plight, I organized and typed the lists from the index cards. When my sister called in the afternoon to ask about Dee and me, I read her the lists. She laughed and said, "You should be able to accomplish everything in the next forty years." We both laughed about that, but I insisted that I could accomplish everything on my lists in just a few years. Then I began in earnest to complete this diary . . . hoping to get it published so that others could learn from our experiences. I also wrote checks, did the books, organized Christmas cards, made plans for the coming winter, and caught up with other pressing items. I took time to call several friends and made plans to go out to dinner with them.

SATURDAY, JANUARY 3, 2015 ॐ

The cook came at nine this morning to make meals but left because her contract was to cook for Dee, not me. I made my own lunch and called the hospital to find out about Dee. Their report was good. Relieved, I worked on the diary for a while, watched football in the afternoon, and went out to dinner with friends in the evening. I did my best not to think about Dee's situation.

MONDAY, JANUARY 5, 2015 ॐ

A week has passed since my son and I took Dee to the hospital for the late-night admission and I am starting to get accustomed to living alone, but not particularly liking it. I went to church yesterday and made an announcement regarding Dee's situation. I asked for prayers for her, and the pastor suggested that prayers for me would also be appropriate. I nodded in agreement but wondered deep down if prayers help anybody with anything. They did not seem to work for Dee. I must have gone to lunch with someone but can't remember.

TUESDAY, JANUARY 6, 2015 ॐ

I drove to the hospital with the two changes of clothes for Dee that the nurse requested over the phone. When I got there the nurse suggested that I go into the large dayroom to sit and talk with Dee. This surprised me because I thought they wanted me to stay away from her so she could be stabilized. The nurse said that visiting Dee shouldn't be a problem, but if it is they would distract her so I could get away. Dee was surprised and pleased to see me. She smiled broadly and gladly embraced and kissed me from her wheelchair. She did not have her usual bright eyes to go along with her smile, and her usually wonderfully fresh breath smelled foul. She looked and acted like a frail old lady, not the vigorous woman I lived with for over fifty years. My heart sank as I realized what they were doing to her and thought, *Couldn't there be something less hurtful?*

I stayed with Dee for about half an hour until the attendants brought her lunch and the nurse took me to a staffing meeting with her, the psychiatrist, the social worker, and the activity director. They reported on the administered drugs and how Dee slept, ate, drank, and so forth. It did not sound good. The nurse said she spits out pills no matter how they are administered. That did not surprise me. They injected antianxiety medications to calm her enough that she would not hit or pinch caregivers. That also did not surprise me. They discussed her new treatment plan, which includes an increased dose of an antianxiety medication in a new form and a small lozenge placed on the tongue that absorbs immediately—so fast that there is no time to spit it out. The lozenge only comes in twice the dosage of the injection but the psychiatrist said this is okay. I did not concur given how Dee acted today and how she previously reacted to increased doses of medication. I told him so, but he replied confidently that I should not worry because her body will adjust to the increased medication. I doubted him because my experience told me otherwise, but I held my tongue. The nurse said she appreciated getting the fresh clothes and adult diapers.

In the afternoon I met my former business partner and his wife at an exhibit at the ASU Art Museum. It felt odd having time to view the exhibit and listen to a video recording by the architect. Dee's attention span had become so short that I could not spend any time enjoying anything of interest to me when we were together.

WEDNESDAY, JANUARY 7, 2015 ❧

I picked up a large bag of adult diapers and a toothbrush and toothpaste before driving to the hospital to deliver them and see Dee. I gave the items to the attendant at the front desk and went to see Dee in the dining area. She again recognized and smiled at me. We embraced and kissed while she remained in the wheelchair. However, she looked and acted even more sedated, like her ninety-year-old mother had in the nursing home in Mesa. I asked the attendant if I could walk with Dee to her room to brush her teeth. The attendant agreed and helped me get her out of the wheelchair and onto her feet. Dee could barely put one foot in front of the other, but we made it to her room with me holding one hand and the attendant the other.

The attendant had Dee remain in the wheelchair in the bathroom as a standard safety procedure while I brushed her teeth. But with her mouth lower than the sink, she drooled toothpaste froth onto the front of her sweater rather than spitting it into the towel that I held beneath her chin. I suspect the foul smell of her breath relates more to the medication than to anything else because the brushing had little effect. We then walked up and down the hallways with Dee saying, "Let's go." I am certain she meant leave the hospital. But I did not bite on her request, so when she tired of walking and we sat down in the common room, she became very agitated and started hitting me. The alarmed attendant jumped up to restrain her. Dee did not hit hard, but such conduct cannot be allowed in front of other mentally disturbed patients.

I had planned to leave at eleven thirty when Dee had lunch but decided to leave earlier to avoid more conflict. The attendant and nurse agreed that this would be a good idea. After my lunch I went golfing to focus on something pleasant rather than driving back to Payson for an Alzheimer's support group meeting. Golf helped me unwind, but I thought a lot about what they were doing to stabilize Dee. I now think of stabilization as something like chemotherapy, where the doctors nearly kill the patient to kill the cancer. I hope Dee comes out of the stabilization process able to remember her friends and function appropriately in social settings without the awful anxiety and anger she experienced so often in recent months.

FRIDAY, JANUARY 9, 2015 ૐ

When I called the nurse after lunch, she informed me that Dee was sitting quietly in her room and had slept well, taken a shower, and allowed the aides to dress her without any problems. Thankful for the good news, I took down and put away the interior Christmas decorations, wondering if I would ever again go into the woods to harvest a Christmas tree. I have a strange feeling of emptiness.

TUESDAY, JANUARY 13, 2015 ૐ

After spending the past few days catching up, I got up early this morning to attend a staffing meeting at the hospital to discuss next steps. They were running late so I went to the common room and found Dee sleeping soundly in a wheelchair with her head bobbing back and forth. She woke up briefly when I spoke to her and greeted me with a little smile before falling back asleep. She did not wake up for the remainder of the half hour while I sat with my arm around her shoulders or rubbed her back. She was completely out.

Everyone at the staffing meeting said that Dee responded well to the new medications and is now easy to care for.

"I hope her condition this morning is not what you are talking about," I stated.

They assured me that this was not usual and that perhaps her sleep medication caught up with her and they might have to reduce it. They agreed to take her off 24/7 care to see if she could sit quietly, participate in activities during the day, and stay in bed at night. If she does well the next couple of days the social worker on her case will contact the memory care facility to evaluate her for placement. I am hopeful and yet anxious about this because I really want Dee to live in this facility.

I went to the common room and looked at Dee. She remained asleep and slumped in her wheelchair. I elected to leave, have lunch, and go to an early afternoon appointment at the Apple Store to learn how to use GPS to navigate around Phoenix. As a trial, I had it direct me to the Rolling

Hills Golf Course and really liked how it worked. However, I could not settle down playing golf until about the fifth hole because I vividly remembered Dee's mom in a sleeping stupor in the nursing home in Mesa. I definitely do not want Dee to remain in this vegetative state the rest of her life and hope that the doctor and staff at the hospital can adjust her medications to a level where she is awake and responsive during the day. It crushes me to see her in such a stupor.

FRIDAY, JANUARY 16, 2015
The parish nurse from our church and her husband visited Dee in the hospital common room in the early evening and said they had a nice visit. Dee recognized them and waved at them to come over to see her. They showed Dee some photos on an iPad and asked the attendant if they could go to her room. The husband sang several songs to Dee in his beautiful deep bass voice and she joined in. After the songs they held hands and the husband, a retired pastor, said a prayer. The wife said they had a wonderful experience.

SATURDAY, JANUARY 17, 2015
Today Dee was awake and reasonably alert in the common room, so I got out our fiftieth anniversary memory book to look at. For over half an hour she moved pages back and forth and pointed at people. When she shook her head to indicate that she could not remember someone, I filled her in. After about forty minutes she got antsy and said, "Let's go," several times. I am sure she meant go home. Instead, I walked her to her room with the attendant. When we got to the room, the attendant asked Dee if she wanted to go to the toilet. I don't recall Dee answering, but the attendant took her into the bathroom and she had a bowel movement.

I heard Dee call out "Mother" several times and give unrecognizable indications of displeasure in the bathroom. When they came out the attendant said, "See, there he is!" She must have assured Dee that I would not go away. We continued to walk around the hallway with Dee repeating "Let's go" several times. When we got back to the common room, I took Dee to her wheelchair and helped her sit down because she seemed tired. Once again she said, "Let's go."

"Honey, it is time for lunch so we should stay. Are you hungry?" I asked.

"Yes!" she said without hesitation.

When her grilled cheese sandwich arrived, I cut it and she grabbed half to eat. With Dee focused on eating, I told the attendant that I would slip out. I had a good experience, especially compared to Tuesday.

SUNDAY, JANUARY 18, 2015 ❧

Another lady friend visited Dee during the lunchtime visiting hours and found her asleep in her room. Dee awoke briefly and smiled, just as she did with me on Tuesday, but immediately fell back asleep and could not be awakened. The lady called and told me about it and said this is not the way she should be stabilized. She was quite upset because her earlier visit with Dee had been much better.

MONDAY, JANUARY 19, 2015 ❧

I called the nurse at the hospital at about eleven to ask about Dee. She said Dee remained asleep in her room, too sleepy to have breakfast, but had taken her pills.

"I think Dee is being overmedicated," I told the nurse.

She checked the chart and said that 1,000 mg of trazodone is not too large a dose for most people. I replied emphatically that Dee responds better to less medication. The nurse said that she would talk to the doctor about the dosage. I asked whether the nurse from the memory care facility had visited. She had not. I felt very bad about Dee's situation.

My younger son called and after lots of discussion convinced me that we are doing the right thing. We just have to make sure they get the medications to the correct dosage. I hope they can and will. I feel like such a jerk for not continuing to care for Dee at home, where she could be alert and happy at times . . . even though she could be agitated or anxious with resulting negative behavior at other times. I called the nurse again after our son's call. She reported that Dee was sitting in the common room asleep in her wheelchair and that the doctor had agreed to decrease her dosage of sleep medication.

"That's a good idea," I told the nurse. "I'll look forward to seeing her awake tomorrow when I come down for the staffing meeting."

TUESDAY, JANUARY 20, 2015 ❧

The staffing meeting was starting late again so I went into the common room where, to no surprise, Dee was asleep in her wheelchair. I sat down beside her and said, "Sweetheart, I am here to see you."

She opened her eyes, smiled at me, and murmured, "I uve ou."

"I love you too," I told her, and started showing her more of our fiftieth wedding anniversary memory book. She was interested and attentive at first, but after a few minutes she had had enough. I asked if she would like to go for a walk. She said yes, so I helped her up from her wheelchair and began to take her for a walk. The startled tech looking after her (and six others because Dee was no longer one-on-one) came over quickly. I told her that we were going to walk around the central core. I did not ask if we could, so she followed close behind, pushing the wheelchair. Dee walked along slowly, holding my hand. She did not grip hard like at home when she was anxious, and her calmness pleased me. We walked around the central core and returned to the wheelchair. When the nurse told me to come to the staffing meeting, I helped Dee into the wheelchair, gave her a kiss, and said I had to go to a meeting. She did not object.

During the meeting they talked about Dee not sleeping at night but rather in the daytime. The nurse suggested that giving Dee sleep medication after nine in the evening made no sense.

Amazed, I said, "Dee always went to bed no later than six thirty because of sundowning, was fast asleep by eight or nine, and slept the entire night without medication."

That the psychiatrist had no awareness of sundowning astonished me, but he did agree to cut her dosage in half and give it to her by six thirty. I thought this was a reasonable compromise. They felt that Dee had calmed down considerably and would soon be ready for release. I felt that they overdid all medications and wished they would release her immediately.

I drove out to see the intake person at the memory care facility to find out when the nurse would evaluate Dee. We discussed the prospects for Dee's admission, but the lady cautioned repeatedly that it would be up to the assessment of the nurse and staff doctor whether or not to admit her. This led to a very apprehensive week on my part wondering what would happen.

WEDNESDAY, JANUARY 21, 2015 ❧

I shared at the support group meeting in the afternoon what they were doing to Dee at the hospital. Apparently it isn't a lot different from the treatment that others receive. Such sharing is good therapy for me. I have so much on my chest to discuss.

THURSDAY, JANUARY 22, 2015 ❧

The nurse at the hospital said that Dee had seven and eight hours of sleep the last two nights. The change in amount and timing of the sleeping pills apparently did the job.

FRIDAY, JANUARY 23, 2015 ❧

I got up late and went to the art class at the community college to tell them that I would like to continue in the class but cannot paint at this time with all the chaos in my life. They had watched Dee deteriorate the last three years and completely understood my situation.

The nurse at the memory care facility called in the afternoon and said she finally got the report from the hospital and was curious about three things: The hospital staff indicated that Dee was not ambulatory, could not feed herself, and slept only four or five hours at night. I responded to the last concern first and told the nurse about the change in dosage and timing of the sleep medication and that Dee had slept seven or eight hours the last couple of nights according to the hospital nurse.

Relative to the first two items, I said Dee could walk and eat by herself before she went to the hospital. I said that the hospital staff put her in a wheelchair from the beginning for fear that she might fall under their watch and assured me that they would get her up at least three times daily to walk around. I doubted that they did this but told her, "I got Dee out of the wheelchair and walked with her around the hallway on Tuesday and she showed no signs of dizziness or anxiety. In fact, she sped up as we approached the common area, saying repeatedly, 'Let's go.' I am sure she can walk without help." I continued, "However, keep Dee away from steps, stairs, and low stools in the middle of rooms because she has a perception problem. Objects appear as much as six inches from their actual location."

I could not explain the difficulty with feeding because with a little help Dee could feed herself.

"I will see Dee on Saturday and check out how she eats lunch," I said.

"Please do. I need to know," the nurse replied.

SATURDAY, JANUARY 24, 2015 ❧

I called my youngest son in the morning to discuss the situation and my fear that the memory care facility might not take Dee because of this latest report from the hospital. He shared my concern and we discussed various things to do. He agreed about checking her out at lunchtime, so I drove to the hospital and walked in at ten thirty to see Dee. The nurse on duty said it was not visiting hours, but I insisted on seeing Dee. I found her awake in her wheelchair watching a murder mystery on the TV . . . a strange program to watch in a psychiatric ward. I walked up to her and she looked up and smiled as I sat down beside her. She was clearly pleased to see me and I was equally pleased to see her, even though her hair had not been washed for several days and her breath still smelled horrible. I think they are less than diligent about washing hair or brushing teeth. I took out an illustrated newsletter and went through it with Dee. At first she seemed interested and to understand what I read. She especially enjoyed seeing her picture and asked about pictures of other people. We did this until they began to serve lunch.

The attendant pushed Dee's wheelchair up to the nearest table and brought her food on a tray. It had a turkey, tomato, and lettuce sandwich on white bread cut into quarters. The tray also held a bowl of vegetable soup, saltine crackers, and a cup of fresh berries as well as three different drinks—a small carton of milk with a paper cup, a bottle of Ensure, and a steaming cup of coffee with a lid—and one small paper napkin around a plastic knife and spoon. Dee's wheelchair did not fit under the low table. Her body and head were at least eighteen inches from the table and even further from the food and drinks on the tray. So I put my hand behind her back and pushed her forward to where she could see the food.

Dee immediately reached out, took the closest section of sandwich, and began to eat. She does not particularly like white bread so she left the top piece on the table and dropped most of the bottom piece on her lap. She grabbed the plastic teaspoon and dipped it in the soup but dropped most of the contents of the very small shallow spoon on her lap on the way to her mouth. I probably would have, too. Twenty inches is a long way to lift a shallow spoon filled with soup.

"Can I help you with the soup?" I asked.

Dee smiled in agreement, so I held the bowl close to her mouth while she spooned the soup into her mouth successfully. She ate nearly all of the soup and the rest of the sandwich, less the white bread. She tried a cracker but did not like it.

"Would you like some milk?" I asked.

"Yes!" she said. So I poured half a cup and gave it to her. She took the cup in her right hand and drank all of it.

Because she never liked Ensure, I asked her if she would like some "milkshake."

"Yes!" she said. So I screwed the lid off the bottle and pulled off the light metallic cover. She clearly would not have been able to do this. She took the bottle and drank about two-thirds of it, then looked at me as if to say, *This is not a milkshake!*

I asked if she would like some fruit but she could not see it from her low-seated position, so I picked up the small bowl and showed it to her. She immediately took out the blackberries with her fingers, one by one, put them in her mouth, and ate them. She looked at the rest of the berries and did nothing until I asked, "Would you like the raspberries, the red ones?"

"Yes!" she said, and promptly picked each one up and ate them. They looked very good to me and she obviously liked them. She just looked at the blueberries.

"Would you like the blueberries too?" I asked. She again said yes and took a few of the small blueberries and appeared to like them, but she had a hard time getting the smallest ones from the bottom of the bowl. I noticed that her fingers were slightly off center and the berries kept sliding out of her grip, probably because of her perception problems. I took the small fork, speared two at a time, and fed the rest to her.

I finally asked, "Would you like some coffee?"

"Yes!" she replied. So I took the lid off the steaming hot coffee and wondered how they expected her to drink it without burning her mouth and/or spilling hot coffee on her lap.

The hospital staff clearly set up everything to make it nearly impossible for a person in a wheelchair with dementia to eat or drink anything. I poured about half of the coffee into the empty soup bowl, then poured some of the remaining milk into the coffee and stirred it with the plastic spoon. Dee took the cup and drank about a quarter of the coffee.

I concluded that Dee could feed herself when seated on an upright chair next to a table, just as she did at home and in restaurants. The situation at the hospital made it impossible for her to feed herself. The food was placed too far away and too high for her line of sight when seated in the wheelchair. The utensils were not appropriate for the task. And there were too many choices of drinks. A person with Alzheimer's cannot be expected to reason or decide on what to drink when offered three choices, especially when she had to open a bottle of who knows what when she can no longer read, remove a tinfoil cover, take a lid off a coffee cup located at least thirty inches away, identify the cup as containing coffee, pour some milk into the cup, stir it, and get it to her mouth when the cup is completely full of very hot coffee.

Is Dee able to feed herself? No! Not if food is presented to her in the way the hospital presents it. Yes, if the food is presented at a table one item at a time with proper utensils. I plan to tell the nurse at the memory care facility this on Monday morning.

The total lack of understanding by the hospital staff about how to present food to people with dementia in wheelchairs amazed and disappointed me. I returned home once again lamenting my decision to have Dee stabilized at this hospital. I feel strongly that they have no idea what they are doing.

SUNDAY, JANUARY 25, 2015 ꙮ

I talked with several of the ladies who visited Dee in the hospital to hear about what they observed and to discuss what to look for at the hospital. I then went to lunch with our usual Sunday group and expressed my concerns about what to do should Dee not be accepted into the memory care facility.

I started thinking about how I could modify our home should Dee have to return. I could have her sleep in a hospital gown, clean her in the shower after bowel movements, and have her use the grab bar to help keep her balance. That would leave my hands free to hold the flexible showerhead to wash off her bottom, and for that matter to clean her body and wash her hair. I could remove the hazard of the two glass doors and cover the raised metal sill with a foam rubber tube to keep it from hurting her feet if she stepped on it. I could remove all of the low end tables from the living room and store them downstairs. I could exchange the love seat upstairs for the couch downstairs to provide Dee a more comfortable place to relax while watching TV or listening to music on the radio.

Now that Dee is much calmer owing to the antipsychotic drug that also treats anxiety and agitation, I could have one lady come at a time (rather than two) to help make lunch and dinner and to feed Dee. I could take care of clothes washing after Dee is in bed so the Dutch door to the basement could be closed when help is here. I could hire one lady to watch Dee for four or five hours every weekday so I could go out to do errands, play golf or tennis, or take a short fishing trip. I could also work on this diary and on a companion biography of my wife, or use this time to clean the basement. Dee would not even need to know that I am home. I could hire one of the ladies to come in early and stay late one day of the week, maybe every other week or once a month, so I could get away for an entire day of fishing, bicycling, hiking, skiing, golfing in the Valley, or whatever.

The big problem would be if I got hurt or became ill. What would I do then? What would Dee do then? Who would take care of her twenty-four hours a day? The imagined arrangement would not work. It would be a disaster. Dee would have to go into an assisted living or nursing home with no prior planning. I did not like this idea. So I called my sister and two sons to tell them about my fears should Dee not be admitted to the memory care facility. They agreed that coming home was not a great option, so we discussed other ideas. The small assisted living home in Star Valley had filled their one vacancy with the wife of one of the men in my Alzheimer's support group. So that is no longer an option. The other assisted living home may work with Dee in her pacified condition.

Another idea occurred to me while talking about a facility in Payson that I previously rejected because we saw only men in the hallway when Dee and I visited the Alzheimer's wing. It did not seem like the right place for my beautiful wife. But our doctor in Payson recently became the medical director of this care center and his very competent nurse practitioner, whom Dee loves, is responsible for all of the doctor's patients in the facility. I decided to talk with the nurse practitioner about her thoughts regarding whether it would be a good fit for Dee. My sons like this idea. I like the idea of not having to drive to the Valley every week or renting a second place in which to live down there, so I hope to explore this Payson possibility. Maybe it is the best option. Maybe it is the answer to prayers that many others and I have offered.

MONDAY, JANUARY 26, 2015 ෨

I called the nurse at the memory care facility early in the morning, hoping to reach her before she went to the hospital to assess Dee for admission to their facility. The owner/director answered the phone so I told him of my concerns about the hospital's report. He tried to get the nurse on the phone but she was on another call so he said to tell him and he would relay the information to the nurse.

I told him about the three items that the nurse called me about. The problem with sleeping at night had apparently been resolved by lowering the dose of sleep medication and administering it earlier in the evening. I told him that Dee had been ambulatory before going to the hospital and that confining her to a wheelchair for a month must have taken a toll. However, I think that her ability to walk could be restored with someone assisting her to strengthen her legs. I even volunteered to come in for a week to assist her. He said they often encounter this problem and have a physical therapist work with patients for a week or two for the same purpose. I explained in detail how the setup at the hospital made it impossible for Dee to feed herself and how I helped her by bringing food close so she could see it and get it with her hands or a spoon.

"The way that your residents are fed will make it much easier for her to feed herself," I told him.

He seemed positive about their ability to handle all of these issues. I also indicated that Dee had been stabilized according to the hospital staff and appeared more relaxed when I visited her. He indicated that the nurse would go to the hospital later that day or the next day to assess Dee.

I called our sons and my sister with the good news. My brother called and I shared this news with him. I want Dee out of the hospital and into this memory care facility before the end of the week and began in earnest to complete all of the paperwork to allow the transfer to take place.

TUESDAY, JANUARY 27, 2015 ॐ♥

I drove to Phoenix in the morning to participate in the staffing meeting at the hospital. They were running late as usual, so I looked for Dee in the common room but could not find her. The person at the desk told me that she was asleep in her room. I went to her room and found her in a very deep sleep, so deep that I could not awaken her.

A nurse came in and said, "She slept barely two hours last night. We could not get her to wake up for breakfast or to take her medicine. The situation remained the same on Monday."

I was wrong thinking that reducing the sleep medication and giving it to Dee earlier solved this problem. I sat silently with Dee for another half hour before the nurse came to take me to the staffing meeting.

The nurse told everyone about Dee's condition the past two days. The therapist claimed that Dee had been very responsive with the afternoon ball-throwing exercises the previous day. The caseworker said Dee is definitely stabilized and ready to be released. She expected the nurse from the memory care facility to visit in the afternoon and wanted them to take Dee before the weekend.

They asked me about my concerns and I brought up my experience feeding Dee in great detail, hoping to give them some idea about how to take care of a person with Alzheimer's disease. I also told them that Dee had walked unassisted only holding my hand lightly on Tuesday, so I know she can walk again if given the opportunity. I similarly expressed that she could sleep all night in a place connected to the outside with light in the daytime and darkness at night. The psychiatrist did not respond positively. He asserted that these changes were a natural progression of the disease. The caseworker felt similarly. I did not argue but felt and still feel strongly that Dee would have none of her current problems if I had not taken her to this hospital.

Stabilized? I thought. *She's been drugged into a stupor!*

My wife did not respond well to the hospital environment or to the antipsychotic drugs because she, unlike the majority of the otherwise healthy patients in the unit with one psychosis or another, was an older person with dementia and they had no idea how to care for her. I was mad as hell but held my tongue.

I feel terribly guilty because this was just like Dee's earlier three-day stay at the health center in Payson, when she became incontinent. These stays result in much reduced capabilities of the woman I deeply love. The medications kill the patient's spirit and competence in order to keep them alive in a reduced state. Is it worth it? I am heartbroken and Dee had her spirit broken. Is it worth it? I will have to wait and see. I still do not know if the memory care facility will take her. I feel so jerked around and unsettled and Dee looks so pathetic, unable even to wake up and give me a little smile. I really dislike the arrogant psychiatrist.

I went back to Dee's room after the staffing meeting to find her on her feet but still asleep, with a large, strong male attendant about to give her a shower before taking her to lunch. I asked him to please wash her hair and told him I would eat lunch in the cafeteria and come back at twelve thirty for visiting hours.

When I came into the common room after lunch, I found Dee dressed with her hair washed, fast asleep in her wheelchair in front of a table. She awakened just long enough to give me a slight smile and for me to say, "I love you!" She repeated very softly that she loved me and fell asleep.

I sat with her for the next hour, propping up her head. She opened her eyes a few times but quickly fell back to sleep. I asked the attendant if she had eaten her lunch. He said no, that she could not stay awake. He indicated that she did better in the shower with the warm water running over her body.

It is so sad! I felt miserable and still do.

I wonder what the nurse from the memory care facility will think when she comes to assess Dee. Will they accept her? I am so totally discouraged and feel like such a failure for not keeping her at home where she could be wide awake during the day, eat her own food with little help, and walk alone all over the house. All of these abilities have been taken from her and they think it is the natural progression of the disease. I know she would be in much better shape if I had kept her at home.

WEDNESDAY, JANUARY 28, 2015 ৶

I waited until eleven this morning to hear from the memory care facility that they had taken Dee away from the disabling hospital environment. I could not stand to wait any longer, so I called the intake person at the memory care facility. It took a while for her to come to the phone because of a staffing meeting. Sitting on pins and needles, I could not imagine how I could have Dee return home with me. I would not know when to ask people to help me because Dee's life pattern is now so different. I have no idea when she will sleep or eat. She would need help every time she tried to walk. What I could do before would not work now.

I neared panic when the intake person came to the phone and said, "We just decided to have Dee come to our facility." I almost cried with relief and asked how soon they could pick her up . . . hopefully by the end of the week. However, the intake person said this was not likely because of the paperwork that must be completed. She said it would be early next week before they would be ready for Dee. She asked me to prepare and send her a long list of items by fax, including the cover sheet I had already filled out, so they could start their paperwork.

I faxed them copies of Dee's driver's license, Social Security card, and all of her insurance cards, two-sided in color, on one 8½ × 11 sheet of paper, plus all of our medical documents. I agreed to bring along the power of attorney and will. The intake person would have all of the admission papers ready to sign.

THURSDAY, JANUARY 29, 2015 ❧

Dee was alone again with no friends scheduled to visit. My feelings of despair for not keeping her home continued unabated. I felt so much like a jerk, ignoring her end-day wishes in favor of following everyone's recommendation to get her stabilized so caregivers could help without fear of getting hurt. I know their arguments make complete sense, but my heart aches for participating in the very serious diminution of my loved one's capabilities and quality of life. I do not know if I will ever forgive myself. I wonder if the staff at the memory care facility can restore some quality to her life.

Meantime, Dee has to spend several more days in the hospital. I saw our nurse practitioner to tell her about Dee's status and my concerns, to check persistent pains in one of my knees, and to advise me on how best to prevent my ears from clogging on my journeys down and up the nearly four-thousand-foot elevation change from Payson to Phoenix . . . one of the side effects of having Dee stabilized and living in the memory care facility in the Valley. Finally, I decided to stay overnight in Phoenix so I could see Dee on both Friday and Saturday to help her walk and eat. I packed for both myself and Dee so she will have new clothes to wear, her own pillow, my mother's handmade quilt for her bedspread, and paintings by her and by me to put on her walls at the memory care facility.

FRIDAY, JANUARY 30, 2015 ❧

I arose early this morning to do my daily yoga exercises before heading to the Valley at nine for the ten thirty meeting with the intake person. I arrived a few minutes late because of rain and dense fog on the way down. The intake person promptly sat me down to sign documents so she could attend an eleven thirty meeting. We got done just in time. I then drove to the hospital to see Dee for lunch. When I got there, she was up but asleep in her chair. I could not awaken her, and the attendant said that she had not eaten breakfast or lunch because she was so sleepy. I sat with her until the end of visiting time and decided to return for evening visiting hours between five thirty and seven. I then visited apartments in the vicinity of the memory care facility.

I organized the trip to visit as many apartments as possible. Several looked like they would work and be in the right price range. I met an attractive young lady at one who had recently graduated from Arizona State University in elementary education. She was looking for an inexpensive studio apartment because she was embarking on her first teaching position at a nearby school. She was so bright-eyed and enthusiastic about the journey ahead of her that she reminded me of Dee when we first met nearly fifty-five years earlier. They took us together to see a studio apartment. The young lady gushed with delight about how it fit her needs perfectly. Her youthful enthusiasm reminded me so much of Dee. I was delighted for her and told her so. However, I was sad in my heart because these personality characteristics had been taken away from Dee. Why did this happen to my wife? Tears flood from my eyes just thinking about it.

I returned to the hospital at six to find Dee in bed asleep. This time I was able to wake her. She smiled and we exchanged kisses. I talked about us for about half an hour before her eyes closed. I sang some of her favorite songs and could see that she enjoyed this by the happy smile on her face. About this time the lady came in that had been her attendant for the first three and last three days. She told me about how lovely but sleepy my wife had been since she returned. Dee awoke again and followed along with the conversation another fifteen minutes.

I stayed overnight at an extended stay hotel in Tempe to see how this might work for me if I spent a couple of nights a week in the Valley. Unfortunately it would cost more than renting an unfurnished apartment near the memory care facility, and I would have the inconvenience of packing and unpacking for every visit.

SATURDAY, JANUARY 31, 2015 ॰♥

I got on the Internet to study reviews of the various apartments I visited. Unfortunately the ones in my price range had some negative reviews. It appears that a lower class of people rent them and bring negatives with them, including drug abuse, noisy pets, and less than stellar cleanliness habits that cause other residents concerns. The more expensive units do not seem to share these problems.

I decided not to look at more apartments and to visit Dee by midmorning in hopes of finding her awake so I could walk with her. I am really concerned that she is losing too much leg strength and balance from sitting in wheelchairs and lying in bed all day. I found her awake in her wheelchair. She saw me, smiled broadly, and waved happily. I signed in, went to her side, and we expressed our love for each other with hugs and kisses. I really needed this. I think Dee did, too.

I told the new attendant that I wanted to walk with Dee. She agreed to let me try and we got Dee to her feet. At first she did not know what to do. It took both the attendant and me to steady and lead her slowly forward before she finally got the idea. We walked around the inner core once. On the second time around we passed a man looking as if he was about to fall forward out of his wheelchair, so the attendant helped him to sit up. But as we walked away the man apparently leaned forward again and fell face-first on the floor. The attendant called for help and soon several other attendants arrived. The man was fairly heavy in build and it was all they could do to get him back into the wheelchair with his limp body. We continued on and gradually Dee became more and more certain about her footing and began to walk faster. This encouraged me. I hope the physical therapist at the memory care facility will be able to get her walking on her own once again.

I asked if we could have Dee sit in a chair at a table for lunch to see if she could feed herself. The attendant agreed. So we sat Dee down with me right beside her. Dee was now high enough to see and close enough to reach her food. She just sat there waiting for someone (me) to feed her. I took the leaves off one large strawberry and gave it to her. She took it in her fingers and took several bites with no further assistance from me. We did the same with the rest of the berries, but with her picking up several from the plate on her own. She did the same with cut up melons and pineapples but left most on her plate until I skewered them on a fork. She took the fork from me a number of times but later I put them in her mouth. I poured milk into a cup and she took the cup and drank from it. I did the same with Ensure. In this case she put down the cup several times but picked it up again to drink until it was gone. She apparently did not like her soup. She took only a few sips using her spoon, then took a bite of cottage cheese but turned up her nose at the taste. She picked up all of the small vanilla wafer cookies and ate them. This encouraged me. I think the memory care facility staff will be able to get Dee back to where she can eat when sitting at a table.

I suggested to the attendant that we walk with Dee before I left for lunch. Along the way the attendant asked Dee if she would like to go to the toilet. Dee agreed to try with my urging but did not have a bowel movement. The attendant then helped me change Dee into a clean shirt. We returned to the common room and walked to the wheelchair with Dee so she could sit in front of the TV. Dee seemed anxious about me leaving but let me go without making a scene. So I guess she is stabilized. Maybe the memory care facility will be able to help her return to normal. I sure hope so!

MONDAY, FEBRUARY 2, 2015 ੭♥

I drove to the hospital in time for the noon visiting hours. Dee had already eaten lunch and enjoyed looking at our memory book for half an hour before losing interest. I then took her for a walk around the ward and helped the attendant change her into a clean blouse. Dee walked much better than before and picked up speed as we circled around the inner core. This took us to the end of the visiting hours. I told her that I was looking for an apartment so I could live near her and also that she would be transferred to a memory care facility the following morning. She wanted to leave immediately. The hospital is such a chaotic place with people with various mental disorders—dementia, bipolar disorder, neuroses, psychoses, schizophrenia—and the people caring for them. A number of people acted out while I was there. It seemed like different nurses and attendants looked after Dee nearly every day and, of course, the lights were on and it was noisy all the time.

I took the elevator to the ground floor, ate a light lunch in the cafeteria, and continued my apartment search. I saw at least eight apartments in the afternoon and liked a small studio apartment at the last place. The lady showing the apartment gave me an application to fill out that night so I could sign up the next day. The apartment rented for $660 per month, the top price I could afford. But the furnishings I own in New Mexico would make it work very nicely.

I headed back to see Dee during the early evening visiting hours. She had just received her meal from an attendant while seated in her wheelchair. I took over the feeding and holding Dee up to the table. Dee immediately picked up the slices of fruit with her left hand. She did the same with the other items. This time the soup cup had a handle intended for sipping rather than spooning. This worked better, but Dee drank less than half of the soup. She drank the milk and Ensure. I showed her more pictures in the memory book before the end of visiting hours. Dee did not resist my leaving, so stabilizing seemed to be working.

I drove north to a hotel near the memory care facility and filled out the application for the studio apartment. While doing this, I received a call from a nurse practitioner at the hospital. She asked if I had noticed Dee's right hand. I replied that I had not but that I had observed her using her left hand to hold things. The nurse practitioner said that the right hand was bent down in an abnormal position all day and they initially thought she might have had a stroke. But because Dee had normal hand strength and nothing else had changed, they thought she might have pinched a nerve in her neck while sleeping. She felt that Dee should have a CT scan of her head and neck to see what had happened. I agreed and a second nurse came on the line to confirm my decision.

The nurse practitioner returned on the line and said that they scheduled Dee for release at ten thirty the next morning. I was glad about this but asked about the scan. She said a physician would read the CT scan in the evening and that the condition would not interfere with Dee's release unless they found something unexpected.

This development did not help my nerves one bit. I have had excess acid and bloating in my stomach ever since Dee went to the hospital. This is getting so old.

Dee went into the hospital with enviable vital signs and came out after a month with a possible stroke, in a near comatose condition, and unable to walk or use her right hand, to stay awake for more than a few minutes each day, or even to show her usual signs of joy or distress. I know this resulted from the poor environment for a person with dementia, including excessive noise, lights on all the time, no loving attention, constant interruptions, inadequate care, and, especially, heavy daily dosages of antipsychotic drugs and sleep medication.

TUESDAY, FEBRUARY 3, 2015 ❧

In the morning after breakfast, I filled out the rental application and made many calls, including one to the hospital to find out what the CT scans indicated. The nurse practitioner told me the neck scan indicated that Dee might have had a ministroke (a transient ischemic attack, or TIA) that could account for the condition of her right hand. She felt that it was not a full stroke because Dee could squeeze her fingers. She also said that the scans indicated that she might have normal pressure hydrocephalus, a condition of the brain and spine involving excessive fluid in the cavities of the brain. The nurse said that this could account for some of Dee's gait and balance problems, urinary incontinence, and even dementia. But she cautioned me not to get my hopes up because generally this is not the primary cause of these conditions. But it did give me another ray of hope.

When I looked up normal pressure hydrocephalus on the Internet, it appeared that it often accompanies Alzheimer's disease and just makes some symptoms worse. It is a condition mainly associated with people in their sixties and seventies and, interestingly, is more common in those with a larger than normal head. Treatment initially includes a spinal tap to remove fluid. The physician checks on the person's gait before and soon after the treatment. If the gait improves, then a more permanent approach includes introducing a long stent into the brain that drains off the excess fluid into the stomach. There are many potential negative side effects to this procedure and its positive effects diminish over time. It appears that my initial hopes were false . . . just like so many have been since 2010.

Memory Care Daily Excerpts ॐ

TUESDAY, FEBRUARY 3, 2015 (CONTINUED) ॐ

I went to the memory care facility to give the intake person a check for the first month's rent and discovered that Dee had just been admitted. They suggested that I accompany her and the nurse to her quarters. I was happy and excited to do this. They let me into the courtyard area and called to the nurse to let me walk along with them. I rushed to the side of Dee's wheelchair and said a happy "Hello!" Dee looked at me without recognition. She was confused and unhappy. I noticed that her right hand hung at her side, bent sharply inward in an unnatural way. She did not lift this hand at any time while I was there. But her mood gradually changed as we walked through the beautiful outside courtyard. She seemed pleased to be outside in the sunlight. I again became hopeful that this might be part of the answer to improving her attitude, behavior, physical abilities, and sleep habits.

Then we came to a high fence with a locked gate separating the main community from the more difficult residents. The nurse put in the gate code and we proceeded to the cottage where Dee would live. This cottage also had a locked entry. This upset me. The unit was beautiful, but not what Dee needed. She was not a criminal to lock up. Again the nurse put in the code to unlock the door. We entered a common room with eight or so residents seated in wheelchairs, upright chairs, easy chairs, and a couch. They seemed happy and alert, with some exchanging small talk with a nurse and an attendant who seemed very pleasant, giving me some sense of relief.

We proceeded into Dee's double room with our beautiful quilt on the bed and our paintings and a photograph of Dee and me on the wall over her bed. That they made this effort pleased me. I talked with Dee about the photo and paintings and she seemed to understand, but I could sense her confusion. Her roommate, a small gray-haired woman with a nice smile, followed us into the room and the nurse introduced her to Dee. She took Dee's left hand, but Dee squeezed back much too hard. The lady pulled away and said sadly, "I don't think she likes me." I tried to assure her that Dee was just confused and upset about being in a strange new place and that she would warm up over time. The lady was not convinced and repeated what she just said. I took hold of Dee's deformed right hand and she squeezed my hand very hard. At least the hand was not paralyzed . . . a small blessing.

It is so unbelievably sad to have Dee experience this. After a bit more comforting talk with her, I excused myself to give the intake person the check, relieved that Dee got out of the hospital before anything more could go wrong.

TUESDAY, FEBRUARY 10, 2015 ❧

I spent this past week moving into the apartment near the memory care facility. I also caught up on household business, including changing a bank account that I had compromised. Mistakes take so much time to correct. I also had a hard time balancing the checkbook for the first time in ages. I eventually discovered that I had added a $5 bank charge instead of subtracting it. There was still a $10 difference that I could not find because I had mistakenly added it a second time. My mind simply cannot focus on the work at hand.

I went shopping to find slacks with the elastic waistbands requested by the nursing assistants in Dee's cottage. I bought four differently colored pairs and decided on size 8 (small) because that is what Dee wore lately. I called Dee in the late afternoon to talk with her. I miss her so much and in so many ways. It took a while to get her on the phone, but when she came on it was amazing. She spoke very clearly. She said hello, and then to my "Hi, Sweetheart, I love you" she said, "I love you too." She said it clearly and with her normal, very sweet loving voice. I had not heard this voice in over a month. Most of the time her speech had been slurred and her voice lacked any tonal quality. This pleased me so much that I looked forward to visiting her the following day. I went to bed early and slept soundly through the night.

WEDNESDAY, FEBRUARY 11, 2015 ❧

I got up very early to get to the memory care facility before Dee's hairdresser was scheduled to arrive, hoping to have the opportunity to instruct her on how Dee likes her hair cut. Unfortunately the hairdresser did not come on schedule. I also found that I should have gotten size 10 slacks to allow more room for the diaper-like underpants needed when Dee is sitting in the wheelchair. I then went to get Dee to take a walk. She was sitting up but asleep in her wheelchair. I tried without success to wake her, so I decided to wheel her out into the sunlight, thinking this might wake her up. It did. I asked the nursing assistant if I could walk with her. She thought it would not work because Dee was so unsteady. I asked if we could try anyway. She agreed but was correct. Dee could not stand up straight because her right leg would not cooperate. Indeed, her whole right side did not work, confirming the possibility of paralysis caused by the TIA or stroke on the last Sunday at the hospital. What a shame that they kept her there so darn long. They did their best to kill her and nearly succeeded.

We went through the locked gate and, holding Dee up on both sides, walked with her about a hundred feet from the cottage, where we sat down on a love seat swing in the partially shaded seating area in the center court. The nursing assistant left to attend to other patients and I put my arm around Dee, whispered sweet nothings in her ear, and massaged her back as she went back to sleep. Her deformed hand hung uselessly by her side. The nursing assistant said that she slept all night but ate very little for breakfast because she was so sleepy.

The physical therapist arrived midmorning and introduced himself. He said that Dee was the same way on Monday and that he could not get her to wake up to do any exercises. We tried to awaken Dee again. She woke up but had a hard time understanding what he wanted her to do and could do no more than two or three repetitions with her legs. Her left leg clearly worked better than her right one. The same was true and even more pronounced with her arms. She could not hold onto anything with her right hand, the one that had always been dominant and strongest. And even while doing these exercises, Dee fell back into a deep sleep.

I now think that Dee had a drug-induced stroke, not a TIA. Her condition is nothing like it had been before whatever it was. And I also think it would never have happened if she had not been over-drugged in the hospital. I was upset with Dee's vegetative state and extremely irritated with the doctor who prescribed so much medication.

The physical therapist could do no more with Dee, so we discussed his continuing schedule and agreed on a time the next Monday morning. I asked how long he would do physical therapy. He said it depended on her progress. Medicare will not authorize continued therapy without progress, and so far there has been none. I told him we would see a neurologist on Thursday morning and hoped she would reduce the medication so Dee could be awake for therapy. I was sure Dee could make progress if awake.

The nursing assistant brought a wheelchair and helped me pull Dee back to the cottage after the therapist left. We went backward because the wheelchairs have no footrests. Because Dee could not raise her feet when asleep, they could get caught under the wheels while going forward. They typically do not keep footrests on the wheelchairs because of the tripping hazard. I saw Dee's feet drag for a few steps but then grabbed her pant legs and held them up to make it easier on her. Dee continued to sleep once inside the cottage, so I decided to go for lunch to get my mind off her sad state. It is hard to see Dee in such a hapless condition. I am a nervous wreck.

I returned to the memory care facility in the early evening to discover Dee still sitting up fast asleep in her wheelchair. This made me so sad and mad about everything. My whole world had imploded. Nothing worked. Indeed, I suspected that Dee was in her last days of life. She was closing down just as her mother did in the last days of her life. I felt miserable and guilty about taking Dee to the hospital. I was culpable in her demise.

I decided to find a hotel nearer to where Dee's neurology appointment would be the following morning so it would be an easy slog to get there before Dee's taxi arrived. I was ready for bed by nine but could not sleep because I felt so guilty for letting Dee be "stabilized." I cried myself to sleep several times during the night. Imagine. A grown man who had not cried for years crying and sobbing like a baby. It was pathetic!

THURSDAY, FEBRUARY 12, 2015 ॐ

I had the hotel call me at seven this morning to make certain that I would be at the neurologist's office before the taxi arrived. I dressed, packed, and ate at the breakfast buffet, then set my phone's GPS to the correct address, checked out, and headed out on time. But the GPS took me to the wrong place. I checked and found that the phone left out the street numbers for some unknown reason. I tried to set it several more times to no avail. Finally, in a panic, I figured out where it should have sent me and headed in that direction. Along the way the memory care facility called me. The taxi driver wanted better directions. Indeed! I did not even know for sure where I was going. When I got to where the office should be, it was not there . . . again. This time, however, I drove into the gas station mentioned in the directions and found a driveway out the back side of the station that led to the office. Strange! I got there earlier than the taxi, so I registered and filled out paperwork until the cab arrived with Dee. The driver and I worked together to get a sleeping Dee into the wheelchair out of the back of the van and then into the office. I completed the paperwork before they called us to another room to have the neurologist see Dee.

The neurologist was taken aback by Dee's condition and her inability to awaken her. "Why is she so sleepy?" she asked.

I told her about the psychiatrist at the hospital prescribing so much medication. She asked whether there was information from the hospital. I told her I had given it to the receptionist when we arrived. The doctor said she didn't have the information because the staff inputs everything into the computer for her to read. So I gave her my copy, which she reviewed quickly.

"Why did they give Dee so much medication?" she asked.

Again I told her what happened at the hospital. She seemed very concerned and said several times that they gave Dee too much medication. I agreed with her and explained how I had suggested less medication at staffing meetings but the psychiatrist did not follow my suggestions.

The doctor tried again but could not get Dee to wake up or respond to anything she asked. I said that neither could anyone else and told her that I could get Dee to open her eyes occasionally but that Alzheimer's had greatly reduced her ability to speak and understand English. I pointed out that part of the reason for coming to see her was Dee's apparent paralysis on the right side from a possible ministroke or stroke. She took note of this but expressed more concern about the irregular but noticeable twitches in Dee's body, fearing that they might indicate some kind of seizure that should be checked out. She wrote prescriptions to reduce the antipsychotic medication by half because it needed to be reduced gradually and to eliminate the sleep medication altogether. She added a small-dose prescription of Depakote Sprinkles for agitation, a net of considerably less medication. The doctor also had her receptionist schedule an EEG in two weeks and another appointment a week later to determine what is going on. I was not thrilled with how long it would take before the next appointment but liked the doctor's genuine concern for Dee's health rather than the disinterested approach of the psychiatrist at the hospital.

Dee remained asleep as we waited for about twenty minutes until another taxi came to return her to the memory care facility. I followed the taxi and helped the driver get her out and into the lobby. I then helped a nurse's aide wheel her to the cottage backward while I followed, holding her feet off the ground by her pant legs. Dee did not awaken the entire journey or when we got to the cottage. I asked them to try to get her to eat or drink something and said goodbye to Dee with a kiss on her cheek. I was really hungry and found a Subway, where I got a sandwich and iced tea. I then drove to the selected apartment complex to see the unit I leased. It turned out to be nicer than expected and I enjoyed thinking about how I would furnish it.

I returned after lunch to the memory care facility to see if Dee had awakened. She had not. I tried to wake her without success, so I eventually gave up and returned to Payson. My sadness about Dee simply overwhelmed me. I felt so guilty for having taken her to the hospital, and then seeing the extreme harm they did to her. She is now so much less capable than when we took her to the hospital. She was alert and generally happy before that. She could walk without assistance. Now she cannot even stand by herself. She had completely normal vital signs before she went to the hospital. Now she suffers from a ministroke or stroke that affects her entire right side. She was awake before. Now she is in a coma.

I think that doctors at the very least should not harm their patients. Dee has been seriously harmed. And I am a basket case. I break into tears whenever anyone tries to console me or tell me that I tried to do what was best for Dee. Maybe so! But I know in my heart that I did the wrong thing to the woman I have loved with all of my heart for nearly fifty-five years. It really hurts to think about it! I feel like I threw her under the bus when she needed me more than at any other time in our married life. I am so ashamed!

FRIDAY, FEBRUARY 13, 2015 ∂❧

This is a suitable day for me: Friday the thirteenth. It seems like my whole life is Friday the thirteenth. Dee's life is, of course, much worse. But why? How could this happen to such a bright light in the world? It is not fair for her, or anyone, to suffer from this terrible disease. And I feel there is no comfort from a higher being, if there is one. The only comfort for her or me comes from loved ones on earth . . . family and friends. If God is present and consoling, it is only through loved ones.

SATURDAY, FEBRUARY 14, 2015 ∂❧

Two friends from our church and I left the house at eight thirty this morning to go to the apartment to unload the furniture. After we finished the unloading the U-Haul truck, I stayed in the apartment, cleaning and straightening the furnishings, then drove to the memory care facility to deliver my valentines to Dee: a Valentine's Day bouquet, four new pairs of elastic waist slacks, and a small white and brown teddy bear. I arrived ten minutes before the planned Valentine's Day party in the recreation room and took all the presents to the cottage to see Dee.

Much to my surprise, Dee was sitting up in a chair and watched as I came in. She seemed confused until I got close and told her that I brought her some Valentine's Day gifts and cards. She recognized my voice, gave me a slight smile, and returned a light kiss as I sat next to her. I gave her a hug and she responded just a little. She took the roses and looked them over carefully before returning them to me. I gave them to the aide to put in Dee's room. I then gave Dee the teddy bear. She held it firmly on her lap for a while with her left hand. She did not use her right hand at all, but I noticed her look at it once, trying to get it to move. Her look showed pure disgust. This was not her body and she knew it.

Dee remained alert while I placed a new pair of reading glasses over her ears and nose and read several Valentine's Day cards to her. I have no idea what she understood, but she paid attention until the last card. Occasionally she seemed to recognize names as I read them aloud. I then took the teddy bear and cards into her room. I put the teddy bear on her bed and placed the cards on her nightstand, along with the vase with flowers. Everything looked very cheerful to me, so I hoped it would have that effect on her each time she entered her room.

The aide then brought Dee into the room to change her blouse because of dribbles on the one she wore. The aide is a tall young woman from Sudan who indicated that she is a Christian and likes her job. She told me she treats it as an important mission for God. The love and gentleness with which she treated Dee pleased me greatly. Dee responded favorably and cooperated as the aide removed the soiled blouse and put on a clean one. She then brought in a wheelchair with footrests so I could wheel Dee to the Valentine's Day party.

At the party the staff served some juice and chocolate brownies, but by this time Dee was asleep and could not be awakened. So I drank some juice, ate a brownie, and participated in the party. The recreation director set up a word game. He printed L O V E across the top of a large piece of brown paper and then four categories down the left side: flowers, cars, movie actors, and towns. The objective was to provide names beginning with the letters above. The people in attendance obviously had memory impairment, but one by one they came up with names. I added a few after they seemed out of appropriate words, hoping that my voice would awaken Dee. She eventually woke up when the matrix was nearly complete. She then listened as each person offered a name and observed the leader as he wrote the names on the matrix. It was a good exercise that everyone obviously enjoyed.

When the party ended and people began to leave, I asked Dee if she would like some juice to drink and she nodded affirmatively. I wheeled her to the table with the pitcher and cups and she drank half a glass of juice, holding it with her left hand. I asked her if she would like a brownie and held it out to her. She took off a small piece with her left hand and ate a little, eventually consuming the small piece and several other small pieces, followed by a few more sips of juice. Seeing her awake and able to respond to what was going on around her made me feel much better than I had the entire week. I had been completely devastated and forlorn about her comatose condition. Taking her off so much medication seemed to have a beneficial effect. I am now hopeful that she will be awake to attend their church service tomorrow afternoon. I drove home feeling better and more hopeful as I planned to attend the Valentine's dinner at our church. Many people at the dinner asked about Dee and I told them about her progress. I drove the truck home for the night and plan to return it in the morning.

SUNDAY, FEBRUARY 15, 2015 ❧

I returned the U-Haul truck to the dealer after breakfast and left it parked in their yard. I then packed everything that the apartment still needed into the Prius, hoping to get this done in time to attend early church and hand-deliver our annual Groundhog Day card to two ladies who helped Dee a lot over the past few years. I wanted to make certain that I thanked them appropriately. However, as with everything else nowadays, I barely got to church by ten thirty so I had to keep their cards to deliver another day.

I left immediately after church to drive to the memory care facility to see if Dee was ready for church. She was awake and appeared happy to see me. I wheeled her to the church service in the recreation room. An attractive middle-aged woman greeted us and directed us to a place to sit to participate in the service. She also led the group in several familiar hymns. Previously Dee would have sung loudly and beautifully along with the others in attendance. Today Dee made no effort to sing, even though others around us were doing their best, including me. She showed no emotional recognition of the hymns or of me singing next to her. The lady gave a rather long and earnest sermon, quoting scripture as she walked around the room. I thought she did pretty well, although I remember nothing that she said. Dee watched her the entire time as if listening but again gave no indication of understanding anything. An old man pastor sitting in front followed the lady with a brief sermon on another topic. I could only think about how Dee used to love church and participate actively in everything. The lady came over to us after the service and invited us to come again. Dee remained completely passive while I thanked the lady and said that I hoped we could return. It broke my heart.

I wheeled Dee back to the cottage, sat with her for a while, left her with the attendants, and drove to the apartment. I spent the rest of the afternoon blowing my nose and straightening furniture in the apartment. I was really suffering from hay fever and happy to get in bed in the early evening because it generally abates once I lie down.

MONDAY, FEBRUARY 16, 2015 ❧

I drove to the memory care facility to assist the physical therapist with Dee and was pleasantly surprised to find her sitting up in a chair in the TV area. She saw and recognized me immediately. I went to her and gave her a hug and light kiss on her cheek. She responded in kind when I said, "I love you," although very quietly.

I asked if she would like to go outside and she replied, "Yes!" I told the attendant, who readily agreed with the plan. Outside, I wheeled Dee around the very pleasant courtyard until the physical therapist arrived. He was happy to see Dee awake. We worked together to give her legs and arms the therapy needed to restore their functionality. Dee had difficulty starting each exercise but once she got the idea did double the number of exercises that he asked for. He was pleased and so was I. We were seeing some light at the end of the tunnel, so to speak. Dee was pleased as we both praised her efforts.

I stayed on with Dee after the therapist left and called her very close friend to tell her the good news and have Dee speak to her. Dee immediately recognized her picture and voice on the phone. She also responded clearly to questions and comments and smiled broadly as she spoke with her good friend. This development was so hopeful. I really think that Dee is coming out of her semicomatose state.

TUESDAY, FEBRUARY 17, 2015 ୧ᵥ

I got up early to drive to the Valley for a doctor's appointment to look into how to keep my ears from clogging while driving between Payson and Phoenix. The doctor had several good ideas and gave me a prescription and recommendations on over-the-counter drugs to combat the differential pressure issues. I also complained about the hay fever that he could readily observe because I was constantly blowing my nose.

I drove to the memory care facility looking forward to seeing Dee awake again, certain that by now the drugs from the hospital had worn off. Wrong again! This time Dee slept sitting in her wheelchair. She had been out all day. I could not awaken her even by taking her into the garden and walking around. I brought along some small tweezers to pluck hairs that had grown long on her chin without her constant care, so I sat beside her in the shaded seating area and plucked them out. Even that did not awaken her.

The recreation director came by and invited us to a get-together in the recreation hall, so I took Dee in but she remained in her trance. Finally, I wheeled her back to the cottage while I began to cough from tickles in my throat . . . something not usually related to hay fever. By the time I got home I was coughing and sneezing regularly. What I thought was hay fever had become a nasty cold that made its way into my chest and head. And I had exposed Dee and others at the care facility to it thinking it was hay fever.

I thought to myself through the evening about how many poor decisions I made this year. I really regret taking Dee to that particular hospital because her capabilities were so diminished by what they did to her. Now I had exposed her to a nasty cold and she does not even have the ability to use facial tissues. I cannot believe how much wrong I have done to her. By the time I got to the apartment I felt bushed and went straight to bed.

WEDNESDAY, FEBRUARY 18, 2015 ❧

I woke up feeling no better than the day before while coughing and sneezing my head off. I called and told the receptionist at the memory care facility that I could not assist the physical therapist because what I thought was hay fever was a bad cold causing me to sneeze and cough incessantly. I asked her to tell the physical therapist to call me about what he finds.

THURSDAY, FEBRUARY 19, 2015 ❧

I called the physical therapist at the memory care facility and he said that he had been unable to awaken Dee and wondered if he should continue trying. I said I would be there the next Wednesday and suggested that we skip Monday and try one more time. I then called the cottage and they said that Dee drank some Ensure at lunch but fell asleep in her wheelchair immediately after. I caught up with a variety of things at home the rest of the day.

Several people visited Dee at the memory care facility during the week and found her in a coma-like condition in which she responded to nothing. She had not eaten anything and drank minimally. One of her friends likened it to closing down before death.

FRIDAY, FEBRUARY 20, 2015 ❧

I called several times to the memory care facility with much the same response. Dee slept most of the time and when awake drank little and ate nothing. Several other friends who visited Dee reported that she had been unresponsive. Another person suggested that she might be in her final stages of the disease and ready to check out. So maybe the end is near.

SATURDAY, FEBRUARY 21, 2015 ঌ

I packed in the morning, cleaned the house, and prepared for Dee's cousins on her father's side to arrive for an overnight stay. I called the memory care facility twice and got similar responses about Dee's condition. The cousins have been good friends of Dee's since she was a child and of mine since our marriage. At dinner we enjoyed talking about past times, particularly times with Dee. We also talked about how my parents had treated them like a son and daughter when they lived in Idaho, even though the man had long hair at that time, during their hippie years he said.

SUNDAY, FEBRUARY 22, 2015 ঌ

We got into our respective cars at nine this morning and drove caravan-style to the Valley, intending to get to the memory care facility just before lunch and hoping to see Dee awake and hungry. Unfortunately she remained in her usual deep sleep and showed no awareness of any of us, keeping her eyes tightly closed during the entire visit. Dee's condition shook up her cousin so much that he broke into tears trying to express his love for her. I sat with her for a long time after they left but with no change in her condition. She did not consume anything all day.

MONDAY, FEBRUARY 23, 2015 ঌ

Today began the same way, with Dee totally unresponsive in the morning and early afternoon. The caregiver in the cottage indicated that Dee had a bowel movement in the morning and urinated once. I went to the movie *Still Alice* in the early afternoon and cried through much of it as it depicted many of the same difficulties Dee coped with in the early stages of the disease. I wondered what Alice experienced in the later stages. Had she ever become anxious and agitated? Had she ever struck out at her husband, daughter, or other caregivers? It appeared to me that the movie never got to the difficult stages of Alzheimer's. It was well done and moving, nevertheless.

I returned to the memory care facility in the late afternoon to see if Dee's condition had changed. To my great surprise and delight, Dee opened her eyes and smiled at me when I gave her a cheery "Hello, Sweetheart!" We exchanged kisses and softly said "I love you" to each other. I was pleased as she kept her eyes open for the next hour and a half. The attendant brought me a glass of juice that I put to Dee's lips and she drank about half of it without stopping, then drank another quarter over time. I hoped that she had reached a turning point for the better.

The attendant asked if I could stay for dinner to see if I could get Dee to eat something. I did and she didn't. I got her to drink another half glass of juice but she would not open her mouth to eat. The meal included meat, potatoes, fruit, and a peanut butter and jelly sandwich, all foods that Dee ordinarily would eat. Through the entire time her eyes were open, including while I walked her around the courtyard in her wheelchair. However, I saw absolutely no expression on her face or in her eyes. They were vacant. It was as if she were in a trance. Perhaps she was. I took her back to the cottage and went to the apartment to get something to eat and get ready for bed because my cold, no longer runny, was up into my sinuses and wearing me down.

TUESDAY, FEBRUARY 24, 2015 ᐫ

I called and told our children, my brother and sister, and several interested friends about Dee's condition. I also shared my concern that Dee may be closing down, calling it quits. Dee said several times in the past how she admired her mother's determination to quit eating and drinking when she neared the end of life. I wonder if Dee decided to do the same. Is she really capable of making such a life-changing decision? I am not certain. But knowing her determination and social awareness, I think she is still capable. I thought of this during the movie when Alice tried to take sleeping pills to end her life. I think Dee's mother simply could no longer swallow. Dee can swallow drinks, but can she swallow food? I do not know. As with everything else, I now feel mostly like a helpless and heartbroken bystander. Should I hope for a change for the better? Should I hope that Dee dies quietly? She has surely suffered enough.

WEDNESDAY, FEBRUARY 25, 2015 ℯ❧

I got up early to meet Dee at the neurologist's office by 7:00 a.m. I arrived before her taxi so I helped the driver get her out and into the office. Dee was awake, but expressionless. We waited in the office until about 7:45, when one of the technicians summoned us into a room set up to perform the EEG. The neurologist wanted to see if mini-seizures had caused Dee's jerking motions so the technician attached many wires to Dee's head and ran numerous tests. Dee just sat there passively as if nothing at all was happening. After a while the technician fetched the doctor, who looked at the results and said there are no signs of seizures. She also saw that Dee's eyes were open, but she did not spend enough time to see if Dee was responsive, which she was not.

We were led back to the waiting room, where I called the taxi to return. It took a long time getting there, so I called again and told the lady at the switchboard that I had an appointment with a physical therapist at 10:00 a.m. so needed to return to the memory care facility. The taxi got to the doctor's office at 9:35 and we had Dee loaded Dee into the taxi by 9:40. I hoped this would be enough time for me to get back for the appointment. It was not, but the therapist remained there waiting for me. I immediately wheeled Dee into a shady spot in the courtyard, but she was completely out. So the therapist and I agreed that there was no sense continuing. The doctor could write another order if or when Dee was regularly awake.

FRIDAY, FEBRUARY 27, 2015 ℯ❧

I got up early and left the house at six this morning to get to an Arizona Alzheimer's Association conference in Mesa in time for breakfast and the opening speech. The conference started with a keynote speaker from the association. He spoke about research findings that vascular dementia sometimes accompanies Alzheimer's disease and can result in ministrokes or strokes like the one that Dee had at the hospital. I quizzed him afterward to see if psychotropic drugs increased the incidence of such ministrokes. He had no answer.

In the first breakout session I heard the mother of the director of the memory care facility talk about meaningful activities for persons with Alzheimer's. She had many good ideas that I want to use with Dee when she gets out of her semicomatose state. I then went to a session about bridging the gap between behavior and communication. The presenter articulated that control of behavior is best achieved by four caregiver behaviors: smile a lot, keep everything simple, go slow at everything, and show (not tell) the person what to do. This results in much more positive behavior by the person with dementia. And always look at your loved one when speaking, even if you are talking to someone else. The person with dementia wants to feel included. She advocated against using any drugs. I cannot agree more.

After lunch, I chose to attend a session titled "Dementia and Psychosis—What We Need to Know." Thankfully a lady leaving the session said that I could take her place, because no other space was available. I heard about minimizing TV, especially violent shows (always on at the hospital), and other distractions. People with dementia need a calming environment. One statement really struck home: "Older people do not tolerate large amounts of medication." I had emphasized this with the young psychiatrist who doubled Dee's dose when she would not swallow pills.

The presenter went on to say that studies of antipsychotic medications showed that they had little benefit for persons with Alzheimer's disease and had significant bad side effects, including tremor, stoop, and shuffle, all of which Dee now had. He then shocked me by saying that a quarter of people with Alzheimer's taking antipsychotics have "significant problems with sedation" and some lose at least a year of life after using these drugs. I was aghast when he said antipsychotics in combination with some sleep medications were a significant cause of death and that extended use greatly increased the chances. Dee had received both types of drugs for over a month at the psychiatric hospital.

After the presentation, I asked the presenter, a research doctor at a different hospital, what he meant by significant problems with sedation. "Putting a person into a comatose condition where they cannot be awakened," he said. This is what happened to Dee. He further told me, "It is almost certain that the combination of antipsychotics and sleep medication will take her life."

I immediately called to find out about Dee. She was asleep and had not eaten anything all day. She remained in a coma, or at least a partial coma that allowed her to wake up periodically. I was really upset as I went to the next session, "A Road Map: Navigating Alternative Choices to Psychotropic Medication." The presenter made it clear that what had been said in the previous sessions was true: people with Alzheimer's disease should not be given psychotropic drugs at all. She emphasized that caregiver behavior is the key to caring for persons with Alzheimer's. I broke out in tears knowing that I had a part in this damaging treatment of my very special loved one. I was completely and totally crushed by what had been done to Dee. I just wanted to help Dee overcome her anxiety, agitation, and consequent aggressive behavior. I did not want to kill her!

I left the conference feeling extremely depressed and drove straight to the memory care facility, hoping to find Dee awake and more responsive. I did not. She was in a deep sleep and had been the entire day. I stayed with her for quite a while, but she showed no signs of waking, even when I repeatedly told her, "I love you, my sweetheart," and cried into her ear saying how much I regretted what I did by agreeing to have her "stabilized." She had no response to anything, so I went back to the apartment, made a light dinner, took a shower (maybe trying to wash off my guilt), and slept fitfully through the night.

SATURDAY, FEBRUARY 28, 2015 ᴁ

I woke up late but very tired, had breakfast, paid the next month's rent, and drove to the memory care facility. Dee was awake at the breakfast table and smiled lovingly at me when I came in but would not eat or drink. She remained awake but unresponsive for a while, then drifted back into a deep sleep and did not wake up through the lunch hour. I went out and got a light lunch for myself and returned to find Dee continuing in a deep slumber. Late in the afternoon I simply had to get out. I drove to a nearby golf course and hit a large bucket of balls and practiced pitching and putting. I went back to the memory care facility to find Dee still asleep. She had not awakened since the morning.

SUNDAY, MARCH 1, 2015 ᴁ

My phone calendar showed me picking up Dee after breakfast and taking her to church. I knew this was not going to happen but hoped and prayed for a miracle, that her strong body and proactive nature would prevail and she would be awake and ready to eat and drink. Dee was awake and sitting in the dining room when I arrived at the cottage at about ten. She smiled warmly at me as I approached her table and said, "Hello, my sweetheart!" We willingly exchanged a tender kiss and "I love you." I then sat down with our fiftieth anniversary memory book and she pulled it toward herself with her left hand. We looked at it together for several minutes, until she suddenly slipped back into a deep sleep.

I asked the caregiver if Dee had anything to eat or drink for breakfast.

"No. Dee has not eaten, but she had a bowel movement and urinated earlier in the morning," she said sadly.

I sat with Dee at the table for a while then wheeled her out into the courtyard, where the sun shone brightly. I again hoped this would wake her up. It did not.

Around noon I brought her back into the cottage so I could leave and get something to eat at the apartment. But on the way I thought, *No, I will not go to the apartment. I will go to McDonald's and get two small cheeseburgers with lettuce and tomatoes, French fries, and a Coke for her and iced tea for me.* Dee always loved this type of meal when she went out on Mondays with the ladies from our church. Maybe she would respond to this offering.

Dee was asleep sitting at the dining table when I got back to the cottage. I sat down beside her and tried without success to awaken her. I then put a small sack of French fries up close to her nose and held it there. Dee obviously smelled them because she sniffed at them and eventually woke up. She looked around blankly until she saw me and smiled.

"I love you very much and have brought a special lunch for us," I said.

She looked at the food on the table and smiled happily. I was so hopeful that she would eat this offering. The lady sitting across the table from Dee smiled and said she wished she could have a hamburger. I pulled out one burger and took a big bite while Dee watched with a happier than usual smile.

"Yum-yum, very good!" I said effusively.

I raised the other burger to Dee's mouth and she smiled at me again but would not take a bite. She gritted her teeth and looked at me smiling, but with a puzzled expression. She was trying to tell me something.

I offered Dee the French fries with the same result. Finally I handed her the cup with Coke in it. She took it with her left hand and raised it to her mouth. She poured a little of the drink against her clenched teeth and grimaced, turning up her nose. She would have none of it. She handed the cup back toward me, but held onto it tightly until I looked into her eyes and at her loving smile. She was trying to tell me something very important.

I took her left hand and told her once more, "Deanna, sweetheart, I love you very much, with all my heart. I always will."

She smiled very sweetly at me and mouthed, "I love you, too." She then drifted into a deep sleep while I shuddered to think what might happen next, beginning to realize what she had just told me.

I stayed with Dee at the table until early afternoon, then wheeled her out to the courtyard and around it several times before heading to the recreation room for the church service by the old pastor and his unnamed but very effective song leader. I sat on a chair beside Dee and held her hand firmly. She responded with a firm grip through all of the singing and preaching that followed, but she did not awaken or show any sign of hearing or understanding. After the service I released my grip and she did the same. She was definitely aware of my presence with her.

I again wheeled Dee around the courtyard and eventually back to the cottage. I stayed with her until about four, when she slumped over to the point that I had the aide put her in bed where she could be more comfortable. I called the cottage after supper and the aide said that he put her to bed and she had not awakened. Seeing no urgent reason to return to the facility, I recorded the happenings of last three days in this diary until about nine, then got ready for bed. By that time I was emotionally exhausted, extremely tired, and sleepy. I was fast asleep by ten.

The cottage caregiver called me at about a quarter to eleven, but I had left my phone on vibrate so I did not hear it. Our oldest son called about ten minutes later, but I did not hear his call either. At about the same time I began to toss and turn in bed. I could not sleep. I tried everything: counting sheep, imagining that I was skiing, thinking about fun times with Dee. Nothing worked.

MONDAY, MARCH 2, 2015 ✒

I tossed and turned all night, until finally at four in the morning I gave up and got up, figuring that I would take a nap sometime later in the day to make up for lost sleep. I went into the kitchen, washed the dirty dishes, then came back to the bedroom to get dressed. I decided to look at my phone and discovered two messages. The first, from the caregiver at the memory care facility, indicated that Dee passed away at 10:40 p.m. on Sunday, March 1, 2015. The second, from our oldest son, confirmed the first call.

I immediately called and awakened our son. He told me the details about how the police needed authorization to take Dee to a funeral home, which he had given them. He suggested that I follow up to make certain that everything happened as the police indicated—to make sure that Dee was taken care of as planned.

I was in shock and denial. How could she pass away? Her grip was still so strong!

Charging Woman ॐ

I came to visit where she lived
She had not eaten
Drank nothing
Was deep in sleep

No one there could awaken her
Nor could I
My words of love
My gentle nudges

But then a hopeful idea came to me
Maybe her favorite foods
Cheeseburger
French fries and Coke

I hastened to buy them and return
She slept as before
My voice held no magic
My touch changed nothing

Held a small bag of fries to her nose
The smell was pungent
Her nose twitched
Twitched some more

She awakened and looked blankly
At the French fries
At the room
At me

Gave me a wonderful loving smile
Recognized me
I said, "I love you"
She mouthed, "I love you, too"

I said, "Sweetheart, I brought a feast"
Cheeseburgers
French fries
Coke

She smiled lovingly at me and the food
I took a bite of my burger
Said, "Yummy, yummy"
Smiled happily

Offered her a bite of cheeseburger
She smiled happily
Clenched her teeth
Would not eat

I suggested, "Maybe the fries"
She smiled happily
Clenched her teeth
Would not bite

Requested, "Please drink some Coke"
She took the cup
Raised it to her lips
Would not drink

Implored, "You need to eat and drink!"
She held the cup firmly
Would not release it
Looked me in the eyes

Hoping for love and understanding
We held the cup
Looked into loving eyes
Her eyes said

"I've had enough and will live no more"
My eyes understood
Her eyes closed
The last time

Charging Woman made her final charge
Snatched victory from disease
Won the last battle
Her way

After the Journey ❧

Gradually I began to accept what Dee had tried to tell me as we gazed into each other's eyes the previous day: *I love you, but I'm going to pass on and go to Heaven.* I cried and sobbed with grief beyond comprehension. The love of my life, my sweetheart, my wife of nearly fifty-four years had passed away, never to wake again, never to give me a hug or kiss, never to give me her wonderful smile. I was bereft . . . totally and completely.

I dressed, brushed my teeth, shaved, ate breakfast, cleaned the apartment, and called the night caregiver about Dee's whereabouts, but he knew almost nothing. He said to call the front office at nine. I then decided to call the funeral home but could not recall which one. I searched through the files in my briefcase and found the record of a call I had made, so I called that funeral home.

The person who answered said they had not received Dee. I nearly panicked. Where was she? I insisted that the person check their records more carefully. The person did and found that Dee was, indeed, in their cold storage facility near the funeral home. I was relieved to know this but shuddered at the thought of my dear Deanna refrigerated. It was not right! The person said to call back after nine to talk with another person about funeral arrangements.

So I continued to do busy work in the apartment and called the funeral home promptly at nine to reach the person with whom I needed to talk. She suggested that I come over so we could decide what to do because Dee had arrived without instructions. This made sense to me because the night caregiver only had instructions as to where she should be taken. I promptly got ready and drove over.

The lady I talked to at the funeral home was very nice and knowledgeable about the various options. I said I want to cremate Dee's body and put the ashes into an ordinary container. (I totally forgot about Dee's wish to give her body to a research hospital.) We do not need an urn. We do not need funeral home assistance with notifying newspapers, writing an obituary, and so forth. We will have services at two churches. The first service, at the United Methodist Church in Payson, will be a celebration of Dee's life. The second service will be in Tempe at University Presbyterian Church, where we will sprinkle Dee's ashes into a small hole in the ground of the memorial garden.

The lady quickly understood what I wanted and settled on a cost to handle the body and do the cremation. I could pick up the ashes when they were ready. I could not see Dee until they cleaned her up and made her presentable without embalming. I agreed to a time and wrote a check for the required amount.

I cried my head off as I drove to the memory care facility (a certain danger to anyone on the freeway and surface roads along the way). I was clearly a distracted driver as I fully realized that my days with Dee, my sweet Deanna, were over. I was alone. So was she . . . in a cold storage facility. It was awful, simply awful.

The receptionist greeted me warmly when I arrived at the memory care facility. She had not received word of Dee's death, nor had anyone else in the front office. I was the bearer of the news. The night shift had recorded Dee's death in the log but left before the front office staff arrived. I brought them up to speed then headed to my apartment.

I began to think of what to do next. My caregiving days were over. Now I had to plan for the funeral and burial. I did not want to do either. I wanted Dee to be alive and with me. If this was not to be, I wanted a wonderful celebration of Dee's life, even though my somber mood would have warranted a very dreary funeral and burial. I was unbelievably sad and discombobulated.

I could not think straight but decided to call the new minister at our church in Payson. Thankfully he answered the phone and was very calm and knowledgeable about funerals, memorials, life celebrations, and the like. We talked about whether to have a celebration very soon or to wait several months. He recommended doing it right away . . . as soon as we could get everything ready. I had no idea how long that would take. He suggested that two weeks would work if I kept at it and that such a short time frame would help keep my mind off my grief. So we agreed on that approach if I could work it out with our children, who must be at both services.

My next task was to tell my family and agree on a date for the services. I spent the rest of the day calling family and discussing possible dates, trying to coordinate with spring breaks. Nothing really worked so we settled on Saturday, March 14, for the celebration in Payson and Sunday, March 15, for the internment at University Presbyterian Church in Tempe. I had designed this church with a memorial garden that my business partner designed. It was the church where both boys were raised and met the girls they married. It was the church in which Dee and I contributed to an interior garden as a memorial to both of our parents. It was our home church.

The celebration of Dee's life was a wonderful occasion, with more than 120 of Dee's friends and family in attendance in Payson and a smaller number in attendance in Tempe.

I SPENT THE REST OF 2015 CATCHING UP WITH THINGS NOT DONE. I RE-ceived copies of Dee's death certificate and provided them to insurance companies so that they could modify their policies. I received and read well over 300 condolence cards with beautifully expressed loving memories of Dee. I sent over 120 letters of thanks to the people who helped me with Dee the past few years and those who sent donations to the Phoenix Alzheimer's Association for research in memory of Dee. The total exceeded $10,000.

I resumed some normal living activities, including housekeeping, gardening, yoga, walking, and other exercise. I participated in several church activities and continued to work on this diary. I resumed work on a love story about our lives that I had begun to write in 2010 when I realized that before long Dee would not be able to answer questions about her life before we met. I continued to go to Phoenix for two or three days a week to do research for a revision and republication of my book on architectural programming that had been out of print for several years. I stayed in the apartment I had leased for a year when thinking I would visit Dee at the memory care facility for years to come. I resumed playing golf regularly and watching sports on TV, went to a few movies, and even attended an opera. I continued going to church and Sunday school each week and out to lunch with close friends afterward. I resumed watercolor, acrylic, and oil painting. In other words, my life returned to some semblance of normality.

Many people asked me how I was doing. At first my response was mixed—some days better, other days worse. Over time I accepted that Dee would not be with me, regardless of how much I missed her, and that I must go on living without her.

As a proactive person, I planned to make the most of my remaining years, resolved to be happy and purposely active. I began telling those who asked, "I am fine, getting on with my life, and looking forward to the years ahead."

Reflections on the Journey ♣

This last stage of Dee's journey was much more difficult and heartbreaking than I could have ever imagined. The decision to have Dee "stabilized" in the psychiatric ward of a major hospital was clearly the worst decision of my life. I forgot advice from a very caring hospice nurse that such a move would be inadvisable . . . that stabilization, if undertaken at all, should be done in an institution dedicated to the care of elderly persons with mental disorders. Furthermore, I learned too late that the combination of antipsychotic drugs and sleep medication are likely to lead to a comatose condition and earlier than normal death for elderly persons with Alzheimer's disease. You cannot imagine the guilt I feel knowing that I contributed to this torturous last stage of my wife's life.

I understand that the loving advice I received from family regarding my deteriorating health was important and appropriate. They recognized that my health was at stake and that if I became ill or died, Dee would be left in a worse state with no loved one nearby to provide the care she needed.

In my grief over moving Dee into someone else's care I made rash decisions, including signing a year's lease for an apartment near a memory care facility before I knew about Dee's condition. I could not accept the fact that Dee was nearing death and was unwilling to let her go.

I am extremely grateful that my loving wife, even in her nearly comatose condition at the hospital and in the memory care center, regained an ability to recognize and love me. This meant so much to me. I continue to admire Dee's proactive nature, even to the point where she took control of how she died. I did not think she had the remaining mental capacity to make such a decision. But I was wrong. She defeated death in her own way.

Advice to Caregivers

1. If your loved one becomes very difficult to care for and starts hurting you or other caregivers, be very careful if you decide to have him or her stabilized. I was not careful enough. First, check for every conceivable medical cause of the agitation and violent behavior. This could eliminate the need for stabilization. If that does not work, search for a neurologist familiar with Alzheimer's disease and willing to work with you at home to stabilize your loved one. This approach will prevent your loved one from being thrust into an unfamiliar hospital

environment. Continue to offer "love medicine," serve the same food, and do the activities that your loved one enjoys. Start with small doses of the drug(s) the neurologist thinks might help stabilize your loved one and modify doses only as needed to produce a calming effect. Be patient if your loved one initially loses capabilities. Hope that the bad behavior will end and adequate functioning will remain.

2. In the Phoenix metropolitan area there is at least one hospital setting oriented toward stabilizing elderly patients with Alzheimer's. If stabilization at home does not work, find one of these facilities if you want your loved one to come out of the stabilization treatment able to function at or near the same level as he or she did before treatment. Is this possible? I'm not certain.

3. I would not advise anyone to place an elderly loved one with dementia in a psychiatric ward of a hospital. The environment is inappropriate, and current research indicates that there are limited benefits and great risks to using antipsychotic drugs on elderly persons with dementia. But if you are being hurt by combative behavior, particularly by a much stronger loved one, you may have to explore this alternative. If so, find a facility that specializes in geriatric care.

4. Beware antipsychotics. The combination of antipsychotic drugs and sleep medication, at least in my wife's case, proved fatal. Perhaps this was a painful blessing for her and me because she died still knowing and loving me and knowing that I felt the same way about her.

5. Research all options. Living with Alzheimer's disease is not a joy for anyone, but I was emotionally prepared to visit Dee frequently for years to help loving caregivers look after her in a memory care facility until she died as a result of the normal progression of the disease. Her early death resulting from inappropriate treatment in the hospital came as a shock. I will always regret my decision to place her in a psychiatric facility. If I had taken time to research all options, Dee might still be alive and feeling loved.

What I Learned ஒ

1. If your spouse's and your work life permit, live near loving relatives. They can provide a family network of support that allows you the time and space needed to retain your own health, both mental and physical.

2. Involve your pastor, deacon, and members of your church in the care of your loved one as early as possible. They cannot change the course of the disease but can help you cope with it and give your loved one the security of interaction with people he or she respects and loves.

3. Dee's illness, especially during the very difficult times, helped me appreciate how very wonderful and loving she had been with me, the boys, and everyone else during our marriage. I had always known and appreciated this, but I could have expressed my love and appreciation to her better and more often. We should not take a person we love for granted.

4. Live life to the fullest each and every day with your loved one. Do all of the important things while you can. Do not assume that life will go on happily until you and your loved one die in each other's arms when you are very old. It is more likely that one or the other will die first or have something unfortunate happen that significantly changes both of your lives so that previous hopes and dreams cannot be achieved.

5. It is important to use love medicine as your primary system of caregiving for a person with dementia. Tell them frequently that you love them. Smile and laugh even when they are difficult. Look at them when talking. Show them what they need to do and go slow.

6. If love medicine by itself does not prevent difficult behavior, it is important to check first for a medical cause (urinary tract infection, abscessed tooth, etc.).

7. If drugs must be used to keep the person calm and noncombative, it is important to avoid antipsychotics, especially in combination with sleep medication.

8. The primary caregiver needs a great deal of personal support, both physical and psychological. Paid health care personnel can provide some physical relief. Family and friends can provide some emotional support. Calls and visits from one's pastor might help prevent the caregiver from losing faith in God. The latter never occurred on my behalf.

Ethical Dilemma ➤

Our American belief system relative to what is an acceptable life and what is not needs some thoughtful reconsideration. When an old dog can no longer use its hind legs to get up to urinate or defecate, most dog owners who love their dog go to a veterinarian to put the dog down. That is the merciful thing to do. When a horse breaks its leg and experience indicates that the chances of the leg healing are slim to nonexistent, the owner will put the horse down. It is the merciful thing to do. But when a human contracts a terminal disease, especially one that causes the person great pain, enough pain that he or she repeatedly asks to be killed, our society forbids us to do this. It would be a criminal act.

However, to drug a terminally ill person to a state of incapacity, a state of oblivion, so the person is alive but incapable of any meaningful existence . . . even to the point where the person is in a partial or full coma . . . is acceptable in our society. Is this the merciful thing to do? Is it acceptable to remove a person with Alzheimer's disease from a supportive and loving environment to one in which all sense of personal identity and security is absent, and then to apply antipsychotic drugs and sleep medications at a level at which the person is constantly disoriented and frightened, or even put into a coma or has a stroke? Is this the merciful thing to do? Has death by this kind of torture become the socially acceptable way to terminate the life of a person with Alzheimer's? Is there a better way? If so, what is it?

6

About Deanna

꒰ꕤ꒱

DEANNA (DEE) VAN DYKE WAS BORN ON MAY 27, 1939, IN SIOUX FALLS,
South Dakota, the first child of Andrew and Margaret Van Dyke. Her
parents and relatives adored the cute, healthy, and happy child. Dee and
her younger sister and brother attended public schools in Sioux Falls
through high school.

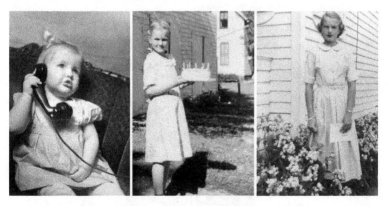

LEFT, *Baby Dee on the phone;* CENTER, *Ten years old;*
RIGHT, *Eighth grade graduation*

Dee majored in elementary education through her junior year at Augustana College in Sioux Falls, after which she took a summer job as a cabin maid and social hostess in Colter Bay, Wyoming.

I met and immediately fell in love with Dee at a folk dancing class in July of 1960 in Colter Bay, and she accepted my marriage proposal after just two weeks of constant courting. We exchanged our marriage vows in her home church in Sioux Falls in March of 1961.

Dee joined me briefly in Philadelphia as I completed a master's degree in architecture. We returned to Sioux Falls immediately after I graduated to visit with Dee's parents, then drove on to San Francisco, where I worked for an architectural firm and Dee taught second grade at a Lutheran school.

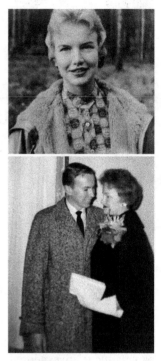

TOP, *In the Tetons, 1960;*
BOTTOM, *Christmas 1960 in the Van Dyke home*

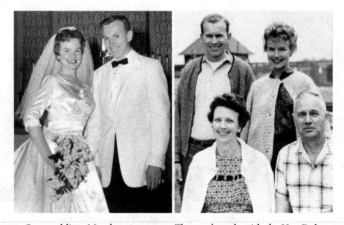

LEFT, *Our wedding, March 1961;* RIGHT, *The newlyweds with the Van Dykes, 1961*

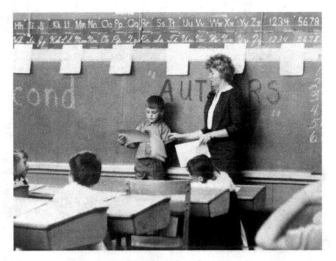

Teaching second grade, 1961

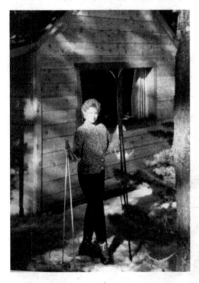

Skiing at Mammoth Mountain, 1962

We loved living in San Francisco and enjoyed many special adventures there, including a trip to Mammoth Mountain, where Dee learned to ski.

The following year we moved to Pocatello, Idaho, where I became an assistant professor of architecture at Idaho State University and Dee obtained a bachelor's degree in elementary education before teaching second grade at two elementary schools. We enjoyed a three-month journey in Western Europe in the summer of 1965 before returning to the States for me to commence studies for a PhD at the University of Pennsylvania. Dee worked at the university library before giving birth to our first son in the spring of 1966, after which she

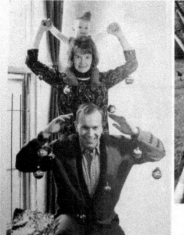
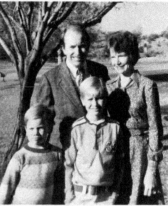

LEFT, *Tree of us, Christmas 1966;*
RIGHT, *The Hershbergers in 1978*

enjoyed life as a full-time mother and having our second son just before I graduated in 1969.

Dee was an incredibly loving wife and mother, helping our boys in every way to become strong, healthy, and reliable people. She used every opportunity to teach them to succeed in any endeavor. She joined the boys and me in every athletic endeavor, including fly-fishing, sailing, and especially downhill skiing, all activities that she never tried prior to meeting me but at which she became very proficient.

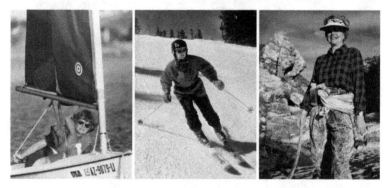

LEFT, *Sailing on Town Lake, Tempe, circa 1980;* CENTER, *Skiing at Sunrise Ski Resort, White Mountains, circa 2008;* RIGHT, *Hiking in the mountains of Arizona, circa 1990*

Dee resumed her career in elementary education after our youngest son began attending preschool, achieved a master's degree in higher and adult education, and taught English as a second language to adults at Cook Christian Training School in Tempe, a Native American theological school. The students at the school gave her the fitting title Charging Woman in a naming ceremony because of her effervescent personality and willingness to overcome any obstacle. I especially appreciated their perceptiveness because Dee never let anything stop her from achieving important objectives in her life. As a natural leader, she enabled everyone around her to succeed.

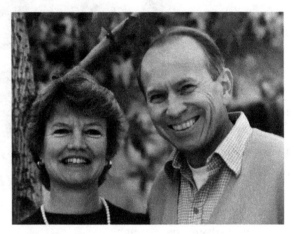

Happy times in Tempe, 1984

Dee's experience at Cook Christian Training School rekindled her lifelong desire to engage in Christian ministry. She subsequently accepted a position as director of the Arizona extension of San Francisco Theological Seminary to provide adult education to Arizona residents for several years. When we moved to Tucson, I became dean of the College of Architecture and Dee served as a development officer at a Christian elementary school and later for the College of Humanities at the University of Arizona. She actively supported me in every aspect of my duties as a college dean, especially helping me with alumni and donor relations.

During this time, Dee pursued advanced studies in theology at seminaries all over the country in order to become an ordained deacon in the Methodist Church. She then served in this capacity in several churches and at Tucson Metropolitan Ministries, a shelter for women and children, while we lived in Tucson. At the same time, both sons obtained undergraduate and advanced college degrees, married wonderful young ladies, and began to have their own families. Unfortunately for us, their careers took them to New Mexico and Ohio. We managed to get together at least twice a year so we could participate with their families as loving and loved grandparents.

We moved to Payson, Arizona, in 2002 to retire and live happily together for the rest of our lives. This worked extremely well from 2005 to 2010, years in which we enjoyed frequent visits with our children and grandchildren, travels all over the world, and bicycling, ski-

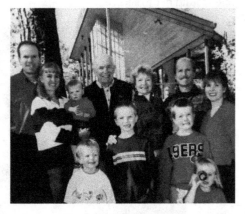

Our family in Payson, 2005

ing, and fly-fishing adventures throughout the western United States.

Our almost idyllic life began to unravel in 2010 as Dee began her journey through Alzheimer's disease. Dee's bright eyes and positive demeanor gradually waned between 2010 and 2014 as the disease took hold and a variety of drugs contributed to a diminished quality of life. A final loving time with our family occurred at Christmas in 2014 when Dee expressed her love to our extended family with gestures

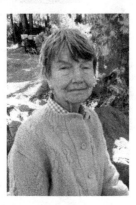

Not feeling great, 2014

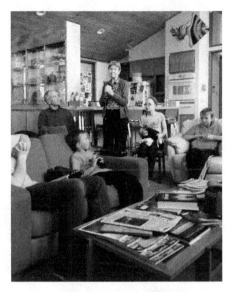

and gibberish in the living room of our home in Payson. Treatment in a psychiatric ward intended to stabilize Dee's negative behavior early in 2015 ultimately destroyed her life completely ... no joy, no beauty, no personality, no Dee, no Charging Woman.

Dee expressing her love for her family, Christmas 2014

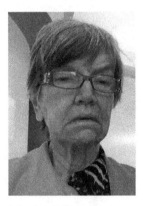

After hospital treatment, 2015

Our love for each other throughout our marriage was unwavering, romantic, passionate, and fulfilling. I loved being married to this intelligent, talented, creative, articulate, exciting, beautiful, religious woman. I loved to talk with her, walk with her, dance with her, and hold her tightly in my arms. I especially loved her radiant smile. We were best friends, confidants, and lovers. If I enjoyed an activity, she quickly learned to do it with me. I did the same with her.

As a natural leader, Dee loved to learn and to share what she discovered with me, our children, and other people. She was a loving and nurturing mother to our two boys and later maintained the same loving relationship with their wives and as grandmother to our six grandchildren.

She is missed and remembered fondly by all of us.

About the Author

BORN IN POCATELLO, IDAHO, IN 1936, ROBERT (BOB) HERSHBERGER AT-tended public schools in Pocatello and earned architecture degrees at Stanford University, the University of Utah, and the University of Pennsylvania. He also earned a PhD at the University of Pennsylvania. He served in the Army National Guard and is a member of the Payson United Methodist Church, AIA Arizona, and the Rio Salado Architecture Foundation. He is a fellow in the American Institute of Architects, past president of the Payson Art League, and a board member of the Friends of Tonto Natural Bridge.

Hershberger taught architecture at Idaho State University from 1961 to 1965, at Drexel University from 1967 to 1969, and as a visiting professor at the University of Texas at Austin in 1976. He served as professor of architecture at Arizona State University from 1969 through 1987 and as professor and dean of the College of Architecture at UA from 1988 to 1996, continuing as professor until he retired in 2002.

Hershberger published numerous articles on how people attribute meaning to buildings and on architectural programming. He also authored the textbook *Architectural Programming and Predesign Manager*, published by McGraw Hill in 1999. In recent years he worked with two collaborators to produce an updated version of this book, titled *Predesign Planning*, published electronically by the National Council of Architectural Registration Boards in 2019.

From 1963 until he retired in 2012, Hershberger practiced architecture, receiving over a dozen design awards for his work. Notable works in

Arizona include the Church of the Palms in Sun City, Alleluia Lutheran Church and the Mill Avenue Rehabilitation Feasibility Study in Tempe, the Longhorn Community Townhouses for Habitat for Humanity in Payson, and his own residences in Tucson and Payson. In addition, he served as western region design consultant for the Disciples of Christ for over twenty years.

Hershberger pursued his interests in watercolor painting throughout his career and has devoted considerable time to watercolor, oil, and acrylic painting since 2004. His paintings are currently shown in the House of Joy gallery in Jerome, Arizona, at the Randall House in Pine, and at the Rim Club and Chaparral Pines in Payson. He participates in several annual art shows of the Payson Art League.

Married for nearly fifty-four years to Deanna (Dee), Hershberger has two sons, Vernon and Andrew, and six grandchildren. He married Sandra Carver in July 2017 and enjoys conversations, attending concerts and movies, watching TV, dining in and out, entertaining, and traveling with Sandy, including an extended honeymoon trip to Europe.

Currently he is completing work on his memoir to be titled *Adventures of an Ordinary Man* and a biography of Deanna to be titled *Charging Woman*. He continues to enjoy taking art classes and workshops, staying in shape, reading, writing, walking, playing golf, downhill skiing, and fly-fishing.

Printed in the USA
CPSIA information can be obtained
at www.ICGtesting.com
CBHW031211100224
4249CB00004B/145

9 781612 497341